Get Through

FRCR 2A: Practice Papers for the Modular Examination

To our families and friends

Get Through

FRCR 2A: Practice Papers for the Modular Examination

Mark Elias
Specialist Registrar in Radiology, Leeds Teaching Hospitals

Rishya Ratnalingam
Specialist Registrar in Radiology, Leeds Teaching Hospitals

Daniel Scoffings
Specialist Registrar in Radiology, Leeds Teaching Hospitals

Michael Darby
Consultant Radiologist, Leeds Teaching Hospitals

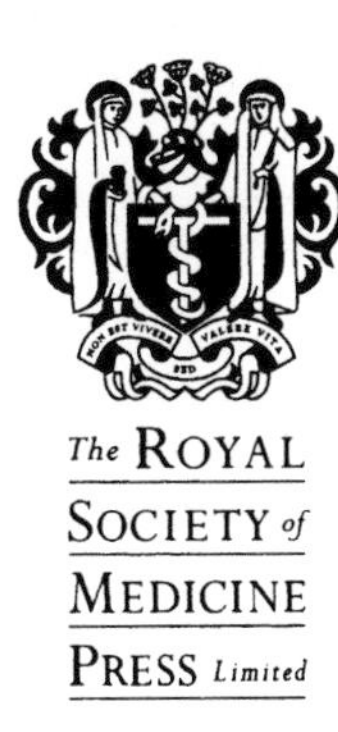

The ROYAL
SOCIETY of
MEDICINE
PRESS Limited

Published by the Royal Society of Medicine Press Ltd
1 Wimpole Street, London W1G 0AE, UK
Tel: +44 (0)20 7290 2921
Fax: +44 (0)20 7290 2929
E-mail: publishing@rsm.ac.uk
Website: www.rsmpress.co.uk

British Library Cataloguing in Publication Data
A catalogue record for this book is available from the British Library

ISBN: 978-1-85315-591-8

Distribution in Europe and Rest of World:
Marston Book Services Ltd
PO Box 269
Abingdon
Oxon OX14 4YN, UK
Tel: +44 (0)1235 465500
Fax: +44 (0)1235 465555

Distribution in the USA and Canada:
Royal Society of Medicine Press Ltd
c/o Jamco Distribution Inc
1401 Lakeway Drive
Lewisville, TX 75057, USA
Tel: +1 800 538 1287
Fax: +1 972 353 1303
E-mail: jamco@majors.com

Elsevier Australia
30–52 Smidmore Street
Marrickville, NSW 2204
Australia
Tel: +612 9517 8999
Fax: +612 9517 2249
E-mail: service@elsevier.com.au

Phototypeset by Phoenix Photosetting, Chatham, Kent
Printed and bound in Great Britain by
Marston Book Services Limited, Oxford

Contents

Preface

In 2002 the Royal College of Radiologists announced changes to the structure of the Examinations for the Fellowship in Clinical Radiology. As part of these changes, Part A of the Final Examination was changed to a modular format with effect from Spring 2004. The following modules are examined:

Module 1: Chest and Cardiovascular (30 questions)
Module 2: Musculoskeletal and Trauma (30 questions)
Module 3: Gastrointestinal and Hepatobiliary (40 questions)
Module 4: Genitourinary, Obstetrics and Gynaecology, and Breast (40 questions)
Module 5: Paediatrics (20 questions)
Module 6: Neuroradiology and Head and Neck (30 questions)

Full details of the structure of the new exam, with a syllabus, are available on the College website (www.rcr.ac.uk).

This book comprises three MCQ papers for each of the six modules examined. As in the exam, 15–20% of the questions in each paper are on radiological anatomy, techniques, and those aspects of physics not examined in the First Examination for Fellowship. Answers score +1 for a correct answer, –1 for an incorrect answer and 0 for no answer. The questions have been written using the textbooks read by UK radiologists in training, supplemented by more up-to-date material from the major radiology journals and specialist textbooks. The answers provide brief explanations, and are comprehensively referenced for further reading.

Acknowledgements

We are grateful to our friends and colleagues in the various departments of radiology in which we have worked during the writing of this book, for providing advice and feedback on questions. In particular we would like to thank Dr Andrew Grainger for his input on Module 2, and Dr William Ramsden for reviewing Module 5.

Abbreviations

CBD	Common bile duct
CSF	Cerebrospinal fluid
CT	Computed tomography
ERCP	Endoscopic retrograde cholangiopancreatography
EUS	Endoscopic ultrasound
FLAIR	Fluid attenuation inversion recovery
FNAC	Fine needle aspiration cytology
FSE	Fast spin echo
Gd-DTPA	Gadolinium-diethylenetriaminepenta-acetic acid
GRE	Gradient echo
HRCT	High resolution CT
IV	Intravenous
IVC	Inferior vena cava
IVU	Intravenous urography
LAO	Left anterior oblique
LPO	Left posterior oblique
MAA	Macro-aggregated albumin
MCUG	Micturating cystourethrography
MRCP	Magnetic resonance cholangiopancreatography
MRI	Magnetic resonance imaging
NEX	Number of excitations
RAO	Right anterior oblique
RPO	Right posterior oblique
SE	Spin echo
SNR	Signal-to-noise ratio
STIR	Short TI inversion recovery
SVC	Superior vena cava
TE	Echo time
TI	Inversion time
TR	Repetition time
TSE	Turbo spin echo
US	Ultrasound

MODULE ONE

Chest and Cardiovascular

Time Allowed: 1.5 hours

Module One: Examination One – Questions

1. **Concerning image processing in digital radiography:**

   a. background subtraction increases contrast.
   b. frame averaging improves SNR.
   c. low pass filtration reduces the effects of blurring.
   d. grey scale processing increases image bit depth.
   e. high pass filtration increases noise.

2. **Regarding thoracic anatomy:**

   a. the parietal pleura extends to the eighth intercostal space in the mid-axillary line.
   b. the SVC enters the right atrium at the level of the third costal cartilage.
   c. the azygos vein drains the first to ninth posterior intercostal spaces.
   d. the left superior intercostal vein is visible on frontal chest radiographs.
   e. the right pulmonary artery passes anterior to the right main bronchus.

3. **Concerning the percutaneous drainage of pleural fluid:**

   a. flow is proportional to the length of the catheter.
   b. flow is inversely proportional to the fluid's viscosity.
   c. maximum flow rate of the catheter is not usually the limiting factor.
   d. intra-pleural streptokinase is a useful adjunct for septated empyemas.
   e. catheters smaller than 14 F are unsuitable for empyemas.

4. **Bronchioalveolar cell carcinoma:**

   a. has an equal distribution between men and women.
   b. is a cause of the 'CT angiogram' sign.
   c. usually presents with diffuse airspace consolidation.
   d. rarely shows pseudocavitation compared to other non-small cell malignancies.
   e. of the solitary nodule subtype is usually central in distribution.

5. **Pulmonary hamartomas:**

   a. often present as a solitary pulmonary nodule.
   b. are usually central.
   c. are well circumscribed.
   d. cavitate in up to 20%.
   e. show calcification at chest radiography in 25–40%.

6. **Regarding Legionnaires' disease:**

   a. lymphadenopathy is absent in most cases.
   b. cavitation is uncommon.
   c. moderate volume pleural effusion is a common finding.
   d. hypernatraemia is a recognised feature.
   e. bilateral pulmonary infiltrates are the usual radiographic pattern.

7. **A 'crazy paving' pattern of ground glass opacification and thickened interlobular septa are seen at HRCT in:**

   a. mucinous bronchioalveolar carcinoma.
   b. lipoid pneumonia.
   c. pulmonary alveolar microlithiasis.
   d. acute respiratory distress syndrome.
   e. alveolar proteinosis.

8. **Pulmonary Langerhans cell histiocytosis:**

   a. is more common among smokers.
   b. presents with a pneumothorax in 10–20% of patients.
   c. has a lower lobe predilection.
   d. typically results in volume loss on the chest radiograph.
   e. is associated with large nodules, which frequently cavitate.

9. **With respect to the pulmonary manifestations of systemic sclerosis:**

   a. it is the connective tissue disease with the highest incidence of fibrosis.
   b. pulmonary involvement progresses more rapidly than in other connective tissue diseases.
   c. aspiration pneumonitis is a feature.
   d. pleural disease is common.
   e. the risk of lung cancer is increased.

10. **In the acute respiratory distress syndrome due to an extrapulmonary cause:**

    a. pulmonary artery wedge pressure is less than 18 mmHg.
    b. the chest radiograph is normal in the first 24 hours.
    c. bronchial dilatation is a frequent finding at CT.
    d. ground glass opacification is the commonest finding at CT.
    e. reticular opacities can persist following clinical resolution.

11. A malignant cause of pleural thickening is suggested by the following CT features:

a. pleural enhancement following IV contrast.
b. nodular pleural thickening.
c. involvement of the mediastinal pleura.
d. circumferential pleural thickening.
e. parietal pleural thickness greater than 1 cm.

12. The following are true regarding usual interstitial pneumonia:

a. the risk of carcinoma is increased.
b. it typically affects the bases.
c. lung volume is preserved.
d. pleural effusions are common.
e. pleural thickening is common.

13. Round atelectasis:

a. has ill-defined edges.
b. is always pleurally based.
c. is always associated with pleural thickening.
d. has a 'comet tail' appearance.
e. is caused by a previous pleural transudate.

14. The following are true of neurogenic tumours of the posterior mediastinum:

a. most such tumours in adults are benign.
b. spinal cord compression occurs.
c. nerve sheath tumours commonly calcify.
d. they are of higher attenuation than skeletal muscle at unenhanced CT.
e. ganglioneuromas are typically broad-based.

15. With respect to CT of mediastinal lymphadenopathy:

a. low attenuation nodes are a feature of Whipple's disease.
b. contrast enhancement is a feature of renal cell metastases.
c. enlarged azygos nodes displace the azygos vein medially.
d. signal characteristics at MRI permit differentiation of benign from malignant causes.
e. paracardiac nodal involvement is common in lymphoma.

16. **Concerning Doppler US:**

    a. pulse repetition frequency (PRF) is inversely proportional to probe frequency.
    b. the Nyquist limit is twice the PRF.
    c. aliasing artefact does not occur with power Doppler.
    d. Doppler shift is increased by increasing the transmitted frequency.
    e. tissue heating is greater with pulsed than continuous wave Doppler.

17. **Regarding the characterisation of cardiac chambers:**

    a. the right ventricle has a muscular conus.
    b. the right atrium has a long finger-like appendage.
    c. the left atrium is characterised by coarse trabeculation.
    d. the left ventricle has a fibrous infundibulum.
    e. the limbus of the fossa ovalis is seen on the septal aspect of the left atrium.

18. **With respect to magnetic resonance angiography:**

    a. fast flowing blood is black on spin echo sequences.
    b. slow flowing blood is bright on spin echo sequences.
    c. MRA underestimates stenoses.
    d. signal intensity depends on TE.
    e. signal intensity is independent of TR.

19. **Features of cardiogenic pulmonary oedema at HRCT include:**

    a. ground glass opacification.
    b. unilateral pleural effusion.
    c. peribronchovascular interstitial thickening.
    d. interlobular septal thickening.
    e. pulmonary arterial dilatation.

20. **Enlargement of the aortic arch on a frontal chest radiograph is a feature of:**

    a. hypertrophic obstructive cardiomyopathy.
    b. ventricular septal defect.
    c. patent ductus arteriosus.
    d. aortic regurgitation.
    e. Marfan's syndrome.

21. Radiographic signs of isolated left atrial enlargement include:

a. a double right heart border.
b. elevation of the left main bronchus.
c. splaying of the carina.
d. inferolateral displacement of the apex.
e. prominence of the anterosuperior cardiac silhouette.

22. The following are seen in hypertrophic cardiomyopathy:

a. spade-shaped left ventricular cavity at MRI.
b. posterior systolic motion of the mitral valve at echocardiography.
c. asymmetric thickening of the interventricular septum.
d. a hyperdynamic interventricular septum at cine MRI.
e. hypertrophy confined to the apex.

23. Regarding Buerger's disease (thromboangiitis obliterans):

a. arterial calcification is a prominent feature.
b. the upper limbs are preferentially affected.
c. disease begins proximally and progresses distally in the limb.
d. skip lesions occur at arteriography.
e. there is no association with cigarette smoking.

24. The following are true of popliteal artery entrapment syndrome:

a. it is more common in men.
b. the posterior tibial pulse is lost with ankle dorsiflexion.
c. it is due to an anomalous course of the lateral head of gastrocnemius.
d. the popliteal artery is deviated medially at angiography.
e. popliteal artery aneurysms occur.

25. Regarding acute traumatic aortic injury:

a. the majority are incomplete ruptures.
b. most cases involve the ascending aorta.
c. it is the commonest cause of mediastinal haematoma.
d. depression of the left main stem bronchus is seen at radiography.
e. post-traumatic pseudoaneurysms are seen in 5–10% of surviving patients.

26. Regarding ultrasound of the deep leg veins:

a. compressibility of a vein excludes the presence of thrombus.
b. acute thrombus is of increased reflectivity.
c. with chronic thrombus, vein walls appear thickened.
d. fixation of valve cusps is a late sign of deep vein thrombosis.
e. in pregnancy, iliac vein thrombosis is more common on the left.

27. **Concerning renal artery stenosis:**

a. catheter angiography underestimates the degree of ostial stenoses.
b. post-stenotic dilatation correlates with the severity of disease.
c. in fibromuscular dysplasia, stenosis is most marked in the proximal third of the artery.
d. peak systolic velocity in the renal artery is increased at Doppler US.
e. intrarenal transit time is reduced at captopril renography.

28. **Following endovascular repair of abdominal aortic aneurysms:**

a. endoleaks can occur via the inferior mesenteric artery.
b. peri-prosthetic gas is a normal CT finding at 2 weeks.
c. most infections present within 1 year.
d. aorto-enteric fistula most often occurs into the jejunum.
e. anastomotic aneurysms are most common proximally.

29. **Post-catheterisation arterial pseudoaneurysms:**

a. show triphasic flow in the pseudoaneurysm neck at Doppler US.
b. can be treated by direct injection of thrombin.
c. older than 7 days are unlikely to respond to US-guided compression repair.
d. will usually thrombose with 20 minutes of compression.
e. of the axillary artery must not undergo compression repair due to the risk of nerve injury.

30. **Concerning inflammatory aortic aneurysms:**

a. the ESR is elevated in most cases.
b. aneurysms are frequently large at presentation.
c. a low-reflectivity halo surrounds the aorta at US.
d. rupture is more common than with atherosclerotic aneurysms.
e. enhancing soft tissue surrounds the aorta at CT.

Module One: Examination One – Answers

1. Answers

a. **True** – removes the same number from each pixel, reducing the effect of scatter.
b. **True** – by the square root of the number of averaged frames.
c. **False** – reduces noise and reduces spatial resolution.
d. **False** – grey scale processing is manipulation of window level and width, bit depth is an inherent property of the imaging system.
e. **True** – this is edge enhancement.

(Farr & Allisy-Roberts pp96–97)

2. Answers

a. **False** – tenth intercostal space in the mid-axillary line.
b. **True**
c. **False** – does not drain the first space.
d. **True** – in up to 10%, forming a 'nipple' on the lateral aortic arch.
e. **True**

(Butler et al. pp5–6 & 127–130)

3. Answers

a. **False** – inversely proportional, it is proportional to the diameter of the catheter.
b. **True** – this is a consequence of Poiseuille's law.
c. **True**
d. **True** – or other thrombolytic agents.
e. **False** – small bore catheters are suitable for empyemas and parapneumonic effusions.

(Tattersall DJ, Traill ZC, Gleeson FV. Chest drains: does size matter? *Clin Radiol* 2000;55:412–421)

4. Answers

a. **True**
b. **True** – mucin secretion causes low density consolidation, highlighting the pulmonary vessels.
c. **False** – the local form of disease with formation of a solitary nodule is the commonest presentation.
d. **False** – it is seen in 50–60% of cases and refers to dilatation of intact air spaces.
e. **False** – peripheral.

(Dähnert pp466–467)

5. Answers

a. **True**
b. **False** – peripheral.
c. **True**
d. **False** – cavitation is extremely rare.
e. **True** – 30% show calcification.

(Sutton pp123–124; Dähnert p489)

6. Answers

a. **True**
b. **True**
c. **True** – in up to 60%.
d. **False** – hyponatraemia due to inappropriate ADH secretion.
e. **False** – usually unilateral.

(Dähnert pp498–499)

7. Answers

a. **True**
b. **True**
c. **False**
d. **True**
e. **True** – 'crazy paving' is a non-specific finding seen in a variety of interstitial-airspace diseases, including SARS.

(Johkoh T, Hoh H, Müller NL et al. Crazy paving appearance at thin-section CT: Spectrum of disease and pathologic findings. *Radiology* 1999;211:155–160)

8. Answers

a. **True**
b. **True**
c. **False** – upper lobes.
d. **False** – increased, unlike most other fibrotic lung diseases.
e. **False** – rarely cavitates.

(Dähnert p498)

9. Answers

a. **True**
b. **False** – slower.
c. **True** – secondary to oesophageal involvement.
d. **False** – uncommon.
e. **True**

(Sutton p199)

10. Answers

a. **True** – this is part of the consensus definition of ARDS.
b. **True** – with preceding pulmonary injury it can be abnormal at an early stage.
c. **True** – associated with ground glass opacification in over two-thirds.
d. **True** – in the acute stage.
e. **True** – with a predilection for non-dependent lung, seen in up to 85% of survivors.

(Desai SR. Acute respiratory distress syndrome: Imaging the injured lung. *Clin Radiol* 2002;57:8–17)

11. Answers

a. **False** – also occurs with benign inflammatory disease.
b. **True**
c. **True**
d. **True** – specificity 100%.
e. **True**

(Müller NL. Imaging the pleura. *Radiology* 1993;186:279–309)

12. Answers

a. **True**
b. **True**
c. **False** – reduced.
d. **False** – rare.
e. **False** – 6%.

(Sutton pp204–206)

13. Answers

a. **True**
b. **True**
c. **True**
d. **True**
e. **False** – exudate.

(Sutton p179)

14. Answers

a. **True**
b. **True** – with extension of a 'dumbbell' tumour into the spinal canal.
c. **False** – this is rare – sympathetic tumours commonly calcify, however.
d. **False** – low attenuation due to their myelin lipid content.
e. **True** – nerve sheath tumours are usually spherical.

(Grainger & Allison pp366–367)

15. Answers

a. **True** – due to fatty replacement, low attenuation also occurs with necrosis.
b. **True** – also melanoma, carcinoid, thyroid, leiomyoma and Castleman's disease.
c. **False** – lateral displacement occurs.
d. **False**
e. **False** – although it is important as a site of recurrence if missed in the radiotherapy field.

(Grainger & Allison pp359–363)

16. Answers

a. **False** – the two are completely independent.
b. **False** – half the PRF.
c. **True**
d. **True**
e. **True** – due to the high PRF and pulse lengths used.

(Dendy & Heaton pp364–373)

17. Answers

a. **True**
b. **False** – the right atrial appendage is squat and short.
c. **False** – coarse trabeculation is a feature of the right atrium.
d. **False** – no infundibulum.
e. **False** – right atrium.

(Grainger & Allison pp675–679)

18. Answers

a. **True**
b. **True**
c. **False** – overestimates the degree of stenosis.
d. **True**
e. **False** – also depends on TR.

(Sutton pp472–481)

19. Answers

a. **True**
b. **True**
c. **True**
d. **True**
e. **True**

(Storto ML, Kee ST, Golden A et al. Hydrostatic pulmonary oedema: High-resolution CT findings. *AJR* 1995;165:817–820)

20. Answers

a. **False** – appears small due to reduced LV outflow.
b. **False** – appears small.
c. **True**
d. **True**
e. **True**

(Chapman & Nakielny 2003 p204)

21. Answers

a. **True**
b. **True**
c. **True**
d. **False** – this happens in left ventricular enlargement.
e. **False** – a feature of right atrial enlargement on a lateral film.

(Sutton p284; Chapman & Nakielny 2003 pp197–199)

22. Answers

a. **True**
b. **False** – anterior motion in systole.
c. **True** – thicker than 14 mm.
d. **False** – reduced septal motion is seen.
e. **True** – occurs in less than 5% and is usually benign.

(Dähnert pp621–622; Haaga et al. p1103)

23. Answers

- **a. False** – calcification is only seen in 10%.
- **b. False** – the legs are affected in 80% of cases.
- **c. False** – disease begins in the palmar and plantar vessels.
- **d. True**
- **e. False** – strongly associated with cigarette smoking.

(Dähnert p616)

24. Answers

- **a. True** – nine times more common in men.
- **b. False** – the pulse is lost with active plantar flexion.
- **c. False** – medial head of gastrocnemius.
- **d. True**
- **e. True**

(Dähnert p643)

25. Answers

- **a. False** – 85% of cases are complete ruptures.
- **b. False** – 88–95% occur at the aortic isthmus, just distal to the left subclavian artery.
- **c. False** – more often due to haemorrhage from the azygos, paraspinal and intercostal vessels.
- **d. True**
- **e. True**

(Dähnert pp616–618)

26. Answers

- **a. False** – acute thrombus has a jelly-like consistency and can be compressed.
- **b. False** – it is of low reflectivity, or non-reflective.
- **c. True**
- **d. False** – one of the earliest signs.
- **e. True**

(Allan et al. pp98–104)

27. Answers

- **a. True** – MRA overestimates stenoses.
- **b. False**
- **c. False** – the proximal third is usually spared.
- **d. True**
- **e. False** – intrarenal transit time is increased.

(Grainger & Allison pp1525–1527)

28. Answers

- **a. True** – also via lumbar arteries (type II endoleaks).
- **b. True** – gas is normal up to 4–7 weeks after repair.
- **c. False** – 70% present after 1 year.
- **d. False** – most commonly into the duodenum.
- **e. False** – most common at the femoral end.

(Haaga et al. pp1671–1676; Dähnert pp607 & 610)

29. Answers

a. **False** – to-and-fro flow is seen.
b. **True**
c. **True** – due to endothelialisation of the neck.
d. **False** – mean of 40 minutes for unilocular and 70 minutes for multilocular pseudoaneurysms.
e. **False** – this has been successfully performed.

(Allan et al. pp82–84)

30. Answers

a. **True** – in 80%.
b. **False** – they present early, due to symptomatology.
c. **True**
d. **False** – less likely to rupture.
e. **True**

(Dähnert p606)

Module One: Examination Two – Questions

1. **With respect to the image receptors used for digital radiography:**

   a. photostimulable phosphors emit light at the same wavelength as the scanning laser.
   b. charge coupled devices require optical coupling with a scintillator.
   c. amorphous selenium directly converts x-ray photons to electric charge.
   d. amorphous silicon is used as a scintillator.
   e. caesium iodide's crystalline structure improves its intrinsic resolution.

2. **The following are true:**

   a. the inferior pulmonary veins run more horizontally than the inferior pulmonary arteries.
   b. the transverse diameter of the right pulmonary artery on a chest radiograph is normally 17–25 mm.
   c. the right superior basal segmental bronchus arises opposite the middle lobe bronchus.
   d. the upper part of the oblique fissure faces medially.
   e. the right upper lobe pulmonary artery arises within the pericardium.

3. **Concerning CT-guided lung biopsy:**

   a. pneumothorax occurs in 20–30%.
   b. it is the gold standard for the diagnosis of pulmonary hydatid disease.
   c. minor haemoptysis occurs in 20–30%.
   d. death due to air embolism is a recognised complication.
   e. it should not be performed as an outpatient procedure.

4. **Lymphangitis carcinomatosa:**

   a. is usually bilateral if secondary to a primary lung tumour.
   b. produces 'beading' of the interlobular septa at HRCT.
   c. is often secondary to an adenocarcinoma.
   d. can mimic pulmonary sarcoid.
   e. is associated with volume loss at chest radiography.

5. **Pulmonary arteriovenous malformations:**

   a. occur more frequently in men.
   b. are associated with hereditary haemorrhagic telangiectasia in 40–60%.
   c. most often occur in the lung periphery.
   d. are multiple in most cases.
   e. are most commonly detected in infancy.

6. **Regarding post-primary tuberculosis:**

   a. most patients are over 65 years of age.
   b. the anterior segments of the upper lobes are the commonest site.
   c. cavitation is a common feature.
   d. pleural effusions are usually small.
   e. mediastinal lymphadenopathy is a common finding.

7. **Inferior rib notching on the chest radiograph occurs in:**

   a. pulmonary atresia.
   b. subclavian arteritis.
   c. neurofibromatosis.
   d. Marfan's syndrome.
   e. Takayasu's disease.

8. **Regarding sarcoid:**

   a. it is characterised by the presence of caseating granulomas.
   b. paratracheal lymphadenopathy is usually left-sided.
   c. a reticulonodular pattern is commonly seen in the mid-zones at chest radiography.
   d. pulmonary fibrosis indicates stage IV disease.
   e. aspergilloma formation is a frequent complication of stage IV disease.

9. **In Wegener's granulomatosis:**

   a. pulmonary nodules occur predominantly in the upper lobes.
   b. renal involvement is a constant feature.
   c. bronchiectasis is a recognised sequel.
   d. pleural effusions occur.
   e. mediastinal lymphadenopathy occurs.

10. **Imaging features of severe acute respiratory syndrome (SARS) include:**

a. 'crazy paving' pattern of lung attenuation at HRCT.
b. mediastinal lymphadenopathy.
c. pleural effusion.
d. cavitation.
e. ground glass opacification, predominantly in the lower lobes.

11. **Regarding *Pneumocystis carinii* pneumonia:**

a. pneumatocoeles occur in most patients.
b. pneumothorax can occur secondary to nebulised pentamidine.
c. lymphadenopathy is a common finding at HRCT.
d. pleural effusions are a characteristic feature.
e. a 'reverse butterfly' pattern of airspace disease is typical.

12. **Malignant mesothelioma:**

a. arises in pre-existing pleural plaques.
b. causes a pleural effusion in 60–70%.
c. causes rib destruction as a prominent feature.
d. commonly calcifies.
e. is associated with cigarette smoking.

13. **Concerning emphysema:**

a. in alpha-1 antitrypsin deficiency, the panacinar type is most common.
b. panacinar emphysema tends to affect the lower zones.
c. bullous change is usually central.
d. bullous change in asymptomatic individuals tends to be basal.
e. it is a cause of 'sabre-sheath' trachea.

14. **The following are true of malignant thymomas:**

a. there is an association with red cell aplasia.
b. they are hypointense to normal thymus at T1-weighted MRI.
c. calcification is seen in most cases at CT.
d. extrathoracic metastases are rare.
e. they are almost always confined within the thymic capsule.

15. **Bronchogenic cysts:**

a. are usually solitary.
b. are usually multilocular.
c. appear as high signal structures at T2-weighted MRI.
d. can mimic left atrial hypertrophy on the chest radiograph.
e. show wall calcification on CT in 30–40%.

16. **The following are true of the NaI scintillation crystal in the gamma camera:**

a. it is doped with thallium to improve durability.
b. it is typically 0.5–1.5 mm thick.
c. the wavelength of emitted light depends on the energy of incident gamma rays.
d. it is hygroscopic.
e. most interactions of 140 keV gamma rays with the crystal are photoelectric.

17. **Concerning the coronary circulation:**

a. the right coronary artery passes between the pulmonary trunk and right atrium.
b. the marginal artery is a branch of the right coronary artery.
c. the left coronary artery arises from the anterior coronary sinus.
d. the left circumflex artery supplies the left atrium.
e. the great cardiac vein runs in the posterior interventricular groove.

18. **Regarding radionuclide studies of the heart:**

a. 50% of the injected dose of ^{201}Tl-chloride localises to myocardium.
b. ^{99m}Tc-tetrofosmin undergoes myocardial redistribution on delayed images.
c. stress images with ^{99m}Tc-MIBI must be acquired within 5 minutes of injection.
d. perfusion defects are seen in syndrome X.
e. pulmonary uptake of ^{201}Tl is increased with left ventricular impairment.

19. **The following are causes of cardiac calcification:**

a. atrial myxoma.
b. myocardial infarction.
c. rheumatoid arthritis.
d. cardiac aneurysm.
e. rheumatic fever.

20. **Regarding primary pulmonary hypertension:**

a. most cases occur in women aged over 50 years.
b. there is an association with Raynaud's phenomenon.
c. a mosaic pattern of lung attenuation occurs at HRCT.
d. the curvature of the interventricular septum appears reversed at CT.
e. peripheral prominence of the pulmonary arteries is seen at CT.

21. The following findings on a chest radiograph are consistent with rheumatic mitral valve disease:

a. straightening of the left heart border.
b. perihilar airspace opacification.
c. enlarged pulmonary arteries.
d. calcification of the mitral valve leaflets.
e. a small aortic knuckle.

22. Regarding Takayasu's disease:

a. rib notching is a recognised feature.
b. the pulmonary arteries are spared.
c. 'skip' stenoses of affected arteries are present at angiography.
d. aortic calcification is a feature.
e. stenoses are more common in the abdominal than descending thoracic aorta.

23. Concerning therapeutic embolisation and its complications:

a. post-embolisation syndrome occurs 24–48 hours after embolisation.
b. the presence of gas indicates abscess formation.
c. hepatic artery embolisation is contraindicated by portal vein thrombosis.
d. renal failure may be caused by necrosis of tissue.
e. pulmonary embolism is a complication of arteriovenous malformation embolisation.

24. Regarding dissection of the thoracic aorta:

a. the chest radiograph is normal in up to 25%.
b. hypertension is the commonest predisposing factor.
c. most are of Stanford type B.
d. transoesophageal US is more sensitive than arteriography in their demonstration.
e. differential enhancement at CT helps determine which is the false lumen.

25. Pseudocoarctation of the aorta:

a. is not associated with congenital cardiac anomalies.
b. causes inferior rib notching.
c. occurs proximal to the origin of the left subclavian artery.
d. causes left ventricular enlargement.
e. does not cause a measurable pressure gradient.

26. **Subclavian steal syndrome:**

a. can occur due to chest trauma.
b. is a cause of ataxia.
c. is more common on the right.
d. is effectively treated by balloon angioplasty.
e. can be demonstrated with colour Doppler US.

27. **Regarding azygos continuation of the interrupted inferior vena cava:**

a. the right gonadal vein drains into the right renal vein.
b. it is associated with polysplenia.
c. the left paraspinal stripe is widened.
d. the right paraspinal stripe is widened.
e. the liver is drained via the azygos vein.

28. **In the assessment of pericardial disease:**

a. small effusions are usually seen posterior to the left atrium.
b. a pericardial effusion with attenuation of 0 HU indicates a transudate.
c. attenuation of 20–30 HU indicates a haemopericardium.
d. both T1- and T2-weighted sequences are needed to differentiate haemopericardium from a conventional effusion.
e. MRI is the technique of choice in investigating congenital absence of the pericardium.

29. **Regarding patent ductus arteriosus:**

a. it is associated with the congenital rubella syndrome.
b. the aortopulmonary window is obscured at chest radiography.
c. the left atrium is enlarged.
d. the ascending aorta is enlarged.
e. calcification of the ductus arteriosus may occur.

30. **Regarding portal vein Doppler ultrasound:**

a. normal flow is hepatopetal.
b. fasting portal blood flow is approximately 50 cm s^{-1}.
c. brief flow reversal is a normal finding.
d. the Doppler angle should be set at 60–65 degrees.
e. portal vein calibre increases post-prandially.

Module One: Examination Two – Answers

1. Answers

a. **False** – the emitted wavelength is less.
b. **True** – often need minification due to their small size (4–5 cm^2).
c. **True**
d. **False** – it acts as a photodiode.
e. **True** – the small crystals act as light pipes.

(Chotas HG, Dobbins JT, Ravin CE. Principles of digital radiography with large-area electronically readable detectors: a review of the basics. *Radiology* 1999;210:595–599)

2. Answers

a. **True**
b. **False** – 8–16 mm.
c. **True**
d. **False** – faces laterally superiorly, and medially inferiorly.
e. **True**

(Butler et al. pp132–140)

3. Answers

a. **True** – 20% is the quoted figure.
b. **False** – hydatid disease is a contraindication due to the risk of fatal anaphylaxis.
c. **False** – haemoptysis only occurs in 2–5%.
d. **True**
e. **False** – studies have shown day case lung biopsy to be safe.

(Chapman & Nakielny 2001 pp188–190)

4. Answers

a. **False** – unilateral in this case, otherwise often bilateral.
b. **True**
c. **True** – breast in over 50%, also colon, stomach, thyroid, cervix.
d. **True**
e. **True**

(Dähnert p502)

5. Answers

a. **False** – twice as common in women.
b. **True**
c. **False** – most often found in the medial third of the lower lobes.
d. **False** – multiple in a third of cases.
e. **False** – the majority are detected in adulthood, 10% present in children.

(Dähnert pp513–514)

6. Answers

- a. **True**
- b. **False** – apical and posterior segments of upper lobe in 85%.
- c. **True** – seen in 50–90%.
- d. **True**
- e. **False** – rare with post-primary tuberculosis.

(Dähnert p533)

7. Answers

- a. **True**
- b. **True**
- c. **True**
- d. **False** – produces a superior marginal rib defect.
- e. **True**

(Grainger & Allison p320)

8. Answers

- a. **False** – non-caseating granulomas.
- b. **False** – right paratracheal lymphadenopathy
- c. **True** – in later disease, upper zone fibrosis occurs.
- d. **True**
- e. **True** – occurs in apical bulla in over half of stage IV cases.

(Dähnert pp522–524)

9. Answers

- a. **False** – nodules show no zonal predilection.
- b. **False** – it is absent in 'limited' Wegener's granulomatosis.
- c. **True** – bronchial abnormalities, including bronchovascular thickening, occur in 40%.
- d. **True** – also pleural thickening.
- e. **True** – also hilar lymphadenopathy.

(Grainger & Allison pp597–598)

10. Answers

- a. **True**
- b. **False** – not described.
- c. **False**
- d. **False**
- e. **True**

(Antonio GE, Wong KT, Chu WCW et al. Imaging in severe acute respiratory syndrome (SARS). *Clin Radiol* 2003;58:825–832)

11. Answers

- a. **False** – occur in 10%.
- b. **True**
- c. **False** – part of the atypical pattern, seen in 5%.
- d. **False** – rare.
- e. **False** – perihilar infiltrates occur in 80%.

(Dähnert pp512–513)

12. Answers

a. **False**
b. **True**
c. **False** – only seen in 15%.
d. **False** – not a prominent feature.
e. **False** – no causative association is established.

(Grainger & Allison p514; Dähnert p505)

13. Answers

a. **True**
b. **True** – worse at the bases, but affects the whole lung.
c. **False** – peripheral.
d. **False** – apical.
e. **True**

(Sutton pp168–172; Dähnert p485)

14. Answers

a. **True** – also myasthaenia gravis, and Cushing's syndrome (due to ectopic ACTH).
b. **False** – isointense on T1- and the same as the surrounding fat on T2-weighted images.
c. **False** – seen in up to 25% of cases.
d. **True**
e. **False** – invades through the thymic capsule in 33–50% of cases.

(Brant & Helms pp320–321; Grainger & Allison pp356–358)

15. Answers

a. **True**
b. **False** – unilocular cysts are more common.
c. **True** – the typical appearance of a cyst.
d. **True** – if subcarinal.
e. **False** – calcification is rare, though the contents may be 'milk of calcium' and appear as relatively high attenuation at CT.

(Grainger & Allison pp364–365)

16. Answers

a. **False** – 0.1% thallium is added to shift the emitted photons into the visible range.
b. **False** – most crystals are between 6 and 12 mm.
c. **False** – the amount of light depends on gamma ray energy, the wavelength is an inherent property of the crystal.
d. **True** – it is hermetically sealed for this reason.
e. **True**

(Dendy & Heaton pp164–165)

17. Answers

a. **True**
b. **True**
c. **False** – posterior coronary sinus.
d. **True**
e. **False** – anterior groove.

(Butler et al. pp164–166)

18. Answers

a. **False** – only 4% localises to myocardium.
b. **False** – it essentially shows no redistribution.
c. **False** – as no redistribution occurs, imaging can be delayed.
d. **True**
e. **True**

(Grainger & Allison pp722–724)

19. Answers

a. **True**
b. **True**
c. **True**
d. **True**
e. **True**

(Dähnert pp583–585)

20. Answers

a. **False** – most cases are seen in young women.
b. **True**
c. **True** – due to regional differences in perfusion.
d. **True**
e. **False** – there is an abrupt decline in pulmonary artery size towards the periphery.

(Dähnert pp643–644)

21. Answers

a. **True**
b. **True** – due to alveolar pulmonary oedema.
c. **True** – with peripheral pruning, due to pulmonary hypertension.
d. **True**
e. **True** – due to reduced forward flow from the left heart.

(Grainger & Allison pp832–833; Dähnert pp636–637)

22. Answers

a. **True**
b. **False** – involved in 50–80%.
c. **True**
d. **True**
e. **False** – stenosis is more common in the descending thoracic aorta.

(Dähnert pp648–649)

23. Answers

a. **True**
b. **False** – can be seen without abscess formation.
c. **True**
d. **True**
e. **True**

(Sutton p456)

24. Answers

a. **True**
b. **True** – in 60–90%.
c. **False** – 60–70% are type A.
d. **True** – sensitivity is 99% for TOE versus 86% for angiography.
e. **True** – in some cases.

(Haaga et al. p1045)

25. Answers

a. **False** – associated with bicuspid aortic valve, PDA and VSD.
b. **False** – no rib notching.
c. **False** – distal to the origin of the left subclavian artery.
d. **False**
e. **True**

(Dähnert p644)

26. Answers

a. **True**
b. **True** – due to vertebrobasilar insufficiency.
c. **False** – three times more common on the left.
d. **True**
e. **True** – reversed flow is seen in the vertebral artery with arm exercise.

(Dähnert pp647–648)

27. Answers

a. **True**
b. **True**
c. **True** – due to an enlarged hemiazygos vein.
d. **True** – due to an enlarged azygos vein.
e. **False** – via the suprahepatic portion of the IVC directly into the right atrium.

(Dähnert pp615–616)

28. Answers

a. **True**
b. **True**
c. **False** – higher attenuation (50–60 HU).
d. **True**
e. **True**

(Sutton pp305–307 & 332–335)

29. Answers

a. **True**
b. **True**
c. **True**
d. **True**
e. **True**

(Dähnert pp640–641)

30. Answers

a. **True**
b. **False** – approximately 18 cm s^{-1}.
c. **False** – it is never normal.
d. **False** – less than 55 degrees.
e. **True**

(Allan et al. p128)

Module One: Examination Three

1. **Concerning digital subtraction angiography:**

   a. subtraction increases image noise.
   b. logarithmic subtraction is performed.
   c. a small focal spot is required.
   d. pixel shifting is used to remove streak artefact.
   e. larger volumes of iodinated contrast are needed than for conventional angiography.

2. **The following are true regarding the PA chest radiograph:**

   a. the centring point is through T8.
   b. an azygos fissure is seen in 0.5%
   c. the left hemidiaphragm is higher than the right in 5%.
   d. the left paratracheal line can measure up to 5 mm.
   e. nipple shadows are poorly defined medially.

3. **Regarding lung scintigraphy:**

   a. breast-feeding women should express and discard milk for 72 hours.
   b. wash-in and wash-out studies are possible with ^{133}Xe gas.
   c. an injection of 500 MBq of ^{99m}Tc-MAA is appropriate.
   d. severe pulmonary hypertension is only a relative contraindication.
   e. ^{99m}Tc-MAA should be injected using the Oldendorf technique.

4. **Features suggestive of benignity in a lung nodule include:**

   a. satellite opacities.
   b. calcification.
   c. no growth in 2 years.
   d. cavitation.
   e. enhancement by more than 20 HU at CT with IV contrast.

5. **Cavitating pulmonary nodules are a feature of:**

   a. Langerhans' cell histiocytosis.
   b. hydrocarbon ingestion.
   c. metastatic malignant melanoma.
   d. *Mycoplasma* pneumonia.
   e. blunt chest trauma.

6. **With respect to pulmonary aspergillosis:**

   a. an aspergilloma is usually associated with pleural thickening.
   b. a fungal ball may be seen to change position within a cavity.
   c. allergic bronchopulmonary aspergillosis (ABPA) causes the 'gloved finger' sign.
   d. ABPA is the commonest cause of pulmonary eosinophilia in the UK.
   e. with repeated episodes of ABPA, the changes are more severe peripherally.

7. **Regarding bronchiectasis:**

   a. bronchiectasis is a reversible dilatation of one or more bronchi.
   b. traction bronchiectasis is associated with interstitial fibrosis.
   c. traction bronchiectasis is most often basal.
   d. HRCT shows marked bronchial tapering.
   e. a 'signet ring' appearance is seen at HRCT.

8. **The following are recognised features of pulmonary asbestosis:**

   a. focal pleural plaques.
   b. hilar lymphadenopathy.
   c. pleural calcification.
   d. pleural effusion.
   e. interstitial fibrosis.

9. **Concerning silicosis:**

   a. fibrosis continues after cessation of exposure.
   b. radiographic changes are most marked in the lower lung zones.
   c. nodules are predominantly seen in the anterior pulmonary segments at HRCT.
   d. there is an increased risk of tuberculosis.
   e. lymph node calcification is seen in most cases.

10. **In the imaging of complications following lung transplantation:**

    a. reperfusion syndrome first manifests 72 hours post surgery.
    b. acute rejection produces septal lines.
    c. acute rejection can cause ground glass opacification at HRCT.
    d. infection is more common in the remaining native lung.
    e. cytomegalovirus infection can cause broncho-arterial fistula.

11. Ground glass opacification at HRCT is a feature of:

a. *Pneumocystis carinii* pneumonia.
b. extrinsic allergic alveolitis.
c. lymphangioleiomyomatosis.
d. alveolar proteinosis.
e. desquamative interstitial pneumonia.

12. Pleural effusions are commonly left sided in:

a. pericardial disease.
b. cardiac failure.
c. hepatic cirrhosis.
d. acute pancreatitis.
e. Meigs' syndrome.

13. Alveolar proteinosis:

a. is associated with leukaemia.
b. is more common in women.
c. causes clubbing.
d. causes cardiomegaly on the chest radiograph.
e. is treated by whole lung lavage.

14. Regarding fibrosing mediastinitis:

a. most patients present with superior vena cava obstruction.
b. the focal type often causes a right paratracheal mass.
c. focal disease is often associated with dense calcification.
d. methysergide is a recognised cause.
e. oesophageal stenosis is a recognised complication.

15. Concerning helical CT for the diagnosis of pulmonary embolism:

a. most emboli can be detected using 'mediastinal' windows.
b. emboli cannot currently be detected beyond third order vessels.
c. tortuous pulmonary arteries are seen with chronic pulmonary embolism.
d. 350 mg I ml^{-1} contrast produces streak artefact in the superior vena cava.
e. beam collimation of 3 mm enables the detection of subsegmental emboli.

16. **Ultrasound:**

   a. has a frequency of 15 kHz or greater.
   b. used in imaging applications has a frequency of 2–15 MHz.
   c. propagates as a transverse wave in soft tissue.
   d. has a velocity independent of the frequency of the transmitted wave.
   e. used in radiology has a wavelength of 10–500 μm.

17. **Regarding angiography of the gastrointestinal tract:**

   a. hyperventilation prior to contrast injection helps reduce motion artefact.
   b. administration of glucagon is contraindicated if hyoscine N-butylbromide has already been given.
   c. a 'sidewinder' catheter is suitable for selective coeliac axis injections.
   d. portal vein opacification occurs 25–30 seconds after injection into the coeliac axis.
   e. 25–45 ml of contrast at 5–10 ml s^{-1} is suitable for the superior mesenteric artery.

18. **With respect to the anatomy of the great vessels:**

   a. the ascending aorta is of larger calibre than the descending aorta.
   b. the left common carotid artery arises from the brachiocephalic artery in 25–30%.
   c. the left vertebral artery arises directly from the aortic arch in 10–15%.
   d. the superior vena cava lies anterior to the right main bronchus.
   e. the brachiocephalic veins receive the inferior thyroid veins.

19. **Arrhythmogenic right ventricular cardiomyopathy:**

   a. results in fibrous replacement of myocardium.
   b. causes thinning of the wall of the right ventricle.
   c. can involve the left ventricle.
   d. results in increased myocardial signal at T1-weighted MRI.
   e. causes right ventricular dilatation.

20. **Cardiac involvement in patients with sarcoid:**

   a. is clinically evident in 20–30%.
   b. results in hyperintense myocardium at T2-weighted MRI.
   c. does not show enhancement with Gd-DTPA.
   d. characteristically causes asymmetric septal hypertrophy.
   e. causes pericardial effusions.

21. If the heart appears small on a frontal chest radiograph, the cause may be:

a. dehydration.
b. hyperthyroidism.
c. Addison's disease.
d. constrictive pericarditis.
e. atrial septal defect.

22. Concerning cardiac tumours:

a. pericardial cysts are more common on the left.
b. most cardiac tumours are malignant.
c. the commonest site for tumour is the left atrium.
d. metastases most commonly arise from the GI tract.
e. heart failure is the commonest manifestation.

23. A right-sided aortic arch:

a. is present in 1–2% of the population.
b. passes to the left of the oesophagus.
c. causes dysphagia when associated with mirror-image branching.
d. gives rise to an aberrant left subclavian artery, which passes between trachea and oesophagus.
e. has a descending aorta which passes through the left hemidiaphragm.

24. The following are true regarding IVC filters:

a. strut perforation is usually asymptomatic.
b. MRI is contraindicated.
c. temporary filters can be left in situ for up to 6 weeks.
d. CT is as accurate as venography in determining the level of the filter.
e. filters must not be placed superior to the renal veins.

25. Regarding syphilitic aortitis:

a. aortic dilatation is usually symmetrical.
b. dilatation usually involves the descending aorta.
c. aneurysms are most often saccular.
d. thin, dystrophic calcification is seen.
e. penicillin is an effective means of treatment.

26. Pulmonary venous hypertension:

a. is usually secondary to left-sided cardiac pathology.
b. results in enlargement of upper lobe vessels.
c. causes Kerley B lines.
d. typically causes small, unilateral effusions.
e. is associated with pulmonary calcification in longstanding disease.

27. The following are true of SVC obstruction:

a. most cases are due to malignancy.
b. there is an association with constrictive pericarditis.
c. presentation with haematemesis occurs.
d. the superior mediastinum is widened at chest radiography.
e. proximal thrombus is a contraindication to stent insertion.

28. Concerning MRI of the heart:

a. endomyocardial fibrosis causes areas of low signal at T1-weighting.
b. marked myocardial thickening occurs with iron overload.
c. atrial dilatation is seen with restrictive cardiomyopathy.
d. myocardial signal is increased in hypertrophic cardiomyopathy.
e. myocardial signal remains abnormal 1 year after the onset of myocarditis.

29. Concerning coarctation of the aorta in adults:

a. an associated patent ductus arteriosus is present in 20–40%.
b. inferior notching of the second to ninth ribs occurs.
c. lobulated retrosternal soft tissue is seen on a lateral chest radiograph.
d. most cases occur in women.
e. balloon angioplasty is the treatment of choice.

30. Ventricular septal defect:

a. results in an enlarged left atrium.
b. causes pulmonary oligaemia at chest radiography.
c. is the commonest form of congenital heart disease.
d. is most often of the muscular type.
e. of the Gerbode type connects right ventricle to left atrium.

Module One: Examination Three – Answers

1. Answers

a. **True**
b. **True** – to take account of exponential attenuation.
c. **True**
d. **False** – to minimise motion artefacts.
e. **False** – less contrast is needed.

(Farr & Allisy-Roberts pp98–100)

2. Answers

a. **False** – T6.
b. **True** – the azygos fissure is present in 0.5–1% of the population.
c. **True**
d. **False** – there is no left paratracheal line, the right line can measure up to 5 mm.
e. **True**

(Francis et al. pp36–50)

3. Answers

a. **False** – this precaution is only required for 12 hours post procedure.
b. **True**
c. **False** – a dose of 100 MBq is typical, less is used for right to left shunts.
d. **True** – as is a right to left shunt.
e. **False** – injection should be slow, the Oldendorf technique delivers a rapid bolus.

(Chapman & Nakielny 2001 pp184–187)

4. Answers

a. **True** – satellite nodules are due to inflammatory disease in 99%, malignancy in 1%.
b. **True**
c. **True**
d. **False** – occurs in tumours.
e. **False** – very suggestive of malignancy.

(Sutton pp108–115; Dähnert pp418–419)

5. Answers

a. **True**
b. **True**
c. **True**
d. **False**
e. **True**

(Dähnert pp420–421)

6. Answers

a. **True**
b. **True**
c. **True** – dilated branching tubular opacities on the PA chest radiograph are due to mucoid impaction in dilated bronchi.
d. **True**
e. **False** – centrally.

(Sutton pp145–149; Dähnert p459)

7. Answers

a. **False** – dilatation is irreversible.
b. **True**
c. **True**
d. **False** – absence of tapering is the most sensitive sign, seen in 80%.
e. **True**

(Dähnert pp464–465)

8. Answers

a. **False** – asbestosis refers exclusively to chronic fibrosis due to asbestos.
b. **False**
c. **False**
d. **False**
e. **True**

(Dähnert pp456–457)

9. Answers

a. **True**
b. **False** – relative sparing of lower zones.
c. **False** – the posterior segments tend to be affected.
d. **True**
e. **False** – seen in 5%.

(Dähnert pp524–525)

10. Answers

a. **False** – manifests within 24 hours, peaks at 4 days and usually resolves by 10 days.
b. **True** – also new/increasing pleural effusion, vascular redistribution, change in the vascular pedicle.
c. **True** – patchy ground glass opacification is the only significant finding after one month.
d. **False** – more common in the transplanted lung due to impaired mucociliary clearance.
e. **False** – invasive aspergillosis can cause broncho-arterial fistulae.

(Grainger & Allison pp578–581)

11. Answers

a. **True** – also other diffuse pneumonias in immunocompromised hosts.
b. **True** – in the subacute phase.
c. **False** – diffuse cysts and a reticular pattern are seen.
d. **True**
e. **True**

(Grainger & Allison p492; Reeder pp516–517)

12. Answers

a. **True**
b. **False** – more common on the right.
c. **False** – right-sided.
d. **True**
e. **False** – right-sided.

(Grainger & Allison pp330–331)

13. Answers

a. **True**
b. **False**
c. **True**
d. **False**
e. **True**

(Grainger & Allison pp601–602)

14. Answers

a. **False** – usually asymptomatic, routine CXR reveals a mediastinal mass. Cough, dyspnoea and haemoptysis may occur.
b. **True**
c. **True**
d. **True** – also secondary to histoplasmosis.
e. **True**

(Dähnert pp475–476)

15. Answers

a. **True** – although small, partial filling defects may be obscured by dense contrast at these settings.
b. **False** – fourth order vessels currently.
c. **True** – also a mosaic pattern of perfusion on lung windows.
d. **True** – therefore tend to use a lower concentration.
e. **True** – as used in the ESTIPEP study.

(Grainger & Allison pp526–529)

16. Answers

a. **False** – 20 kHz or more.
b. **True**
c. **False** – longitudinal wave.
d. **True** – the speed of sound is constant for a given medium.
e. **True** – assuming a speed of sound of 1500 ms s^{-1}, at 3 Mhz the wavelength is 500 μm and at 15 MHz it is 10 μm.

(Dendy & Heaton pp330–332)

17. Answers

a. **True**
b. **False**
c. **True**
d. **False** – 8–14 seconds.
e. **True** – 300 mg I ml^{-1} strength contrast.

(Grainger & Allison pp1166–1168)

18. Answers

a. **True**
b. **True**
c. **False** – 2.5%.
d. **True**
e. **True**

(Butler et al. pp168–169)

19. Answers

a. **True** – also fatty replacement.
b. **True**
c. **True** – septal and left ventricular involvement occurs less commonly.
d. **True**
e. **True**

(Grainger & Allison pp757–759)

20. Answers

a. **False** – it is seen at post-mortem in 20–30%, but only 5% have symptoms.
b. **True**
c. **False**
d. **False** – this is a feature of hypertrophic cardiomyopathy.
e. **True** – although uncommon.

(Grainger & Allison p757; Dähnert p522–524)

21. Answers

a. **True**
b. **False** – cardiac enlargement due to hyperdynamic circulation.
c. **True**
d. **True**
e. **False**

(Chapman & Nakielny 2003 p196)

22. Answers

a. **False** – right.
b. **False** – benign.
c. **True**
d. **False** – lung and breast more common.
e. **False** – pericardial effusion.

(Sutton pp307–309 & 336–339)

23. Answers

a. **True**
b. **False** – to the right.
c. **False** – there is no vascular sling, so no dysphagia occurs.
d. **False** – behind the oesophagus.
e. **True**

(Dähnert pp577–579)

24. Answers

a. **True**
b. **False**
c. **False** – temporary filters should be removed after 2 weeks.
d. **True**
e. **False** – although usually sited infrarenally, filters may rarely need placing in the suprarenal IVC, e.g. for renal vein thrombosis as a source of emboli.

(Haaga et al. pp1682–1683)

25. Answers

a. **False** – asymmetrical.
b. **False** – root/ascending.
c. **True**
d. **True**
e. **False** – surgery is the only effective means of treatment.

(Sutton p313)

26. Answers

a. **True**
b. **True**
c. **True**
d. **False** – effusions are usually bilateral and large.
e. **True**

(Sutton pp288–289)

27. Answers

a. **True** – 80–90% due to malignancy.
b. **True**
c. **True** – due to 'downhill' oesophageal varices.
d. **True**
e. **False**

(Dähnert p648; Grainger & Allison p617)

28. Answers

a. **True**
b. **False** – only mildly thickened.
c. **True**
d. **True** – on spin echo sequences.
e. **False** – signal abnormalities resolve after 3 months.

(Grainger & Allison pp756–759)

29. Answers

a. **False** – coexistent cardiac anomalies are rare with adult coarctation.
b. **False** – the second ribs do not show notching.
c. **True** – enlarged internal mammary arteries.
d. **False** – 80% occur in men.
e. **False** – angioplasty has a high restenosis rate, surgery is preferred.

(Dähnert pp622–623; Grainger & Allison pp948–950)

30. Answers

a. **True** – also enlarged left ventricle.
b. **False** – pulmonary plethora.
c. **True**
d. **False** – membranous VSD in 75–80%.
e. **False** – left ventricle to right atrium.

(Dähnert pp655–656; Grainger & Allison pp790–791)

MODULE TWO

Musculoskeletal and Trauma

Time Allowed: 1.5 hours

Module Two: Examination One – Questions

1. **At MRI of a limb, the susceptibility artefact from an intramedullary nail can be reduced by:**

   a. using a fast spin echo instead of spin echo sequence.
   b. increasing the field strength, B_0.
   c. increasing TE.
   d. orientating the nail parallel to the long axis of B_0.
   e. increasing the gradient field strength.

2. **Regarding anatomy around the ankle:**

   a. the deltoid ligament lies laterally.
   b. the tendon of tibialis posterior lies behind the medial malleolus.
   c. the Achilles tendon shares a synovial sheath with plantaris.
   d. peroneus brevis inserts into the talus.
   e. the os trigonum lies posterior to the talus.

3. **The centring point for:**

   a. a dorsipalmar view of the hand is the head of the third metacarpal.
   b. an AP view of the shoulder is the humeral head.
   c. a lateral view of the elbow is the lateral epicondyle.
   d. an AP view of the hips is 5 cm above the superior border of the symphysis pubis.
   e. an AP view of the ankle is 2.5 cm above the joint line.

4. **Concerning facial injuries:**

   a. the nasal bones are the most commonly fractured.
   b. the zygomaticomaxillary complex (ZMC) fracture involves the inferior orbital rim.
   c. isolated fractures of the maxillary antra are uncommon.
   d. the LeFort I fracture is a transverse fracture of the maxillary alveolus.
   e. a LeFort III fracture is typically associated with a ZMC fracture on the side of impact.

5. **Concerning injuries of the cervical spine:**

   a. wedge compression fractures disrupt the posterior ligamentous complex.
   b. wedge compression fractures are stable injuries.
   c. clay shoveler's fractures are characteristically comminuted.
   d. the fragment of a flexion teardrop fracture arises from the anterosuperior vertebral body.
   e. unilateral interfacetal dislocation is an unstable injury.

6. **Regarding trauma to the clavicle:**

   a. it is the most frequent fracture site in childhood.
   b. the medial end is usually elevated with complete fractures.
   c. the lateral third is most often affected.
   d. non-union is common.
   e. associated injury to the subclavian vein is more common than to the artery.

7. **Concerning carpal instability:**

   a. scapholunate dissociation is the commonest form.
   b. the scapholunate angle is less than 30 degrees in dorsal intercalated segmental instability (DISI).
   c. the scapholunate angle is more than 80 degrees in ventral intercalated segmental instability (VISI).
   d. DISI is more common than VISI.
   e. most cases of DISI and VISI are associated with a scaphoid fracture.

8. **With respect to fractures of the patella:**

   a. the majority are transverse.
   b. fragments are often widely separated with a transverse fracture.
   c. avulsion fractures are best seen on a skyline view.
   d. osteochondral fractures arise from the medial facet.
   e. osteochondral fractures are best seen on an axial view.

9. **Regarding anterior dislocation of the shoulder:**

   a. the humeral head lies inferior and lateral to the glenoid on an AP film.
   b. the presence of a Hill–Sachs defect indicates recurrent previous dislocations.
   c. a Hill–Sachs defect affects the inferior glenoid.
   d. Bankart lesions are more common than Hill–Sachs defects.
   e. it accounts for 50–75% of shoulder dislocations.

10. **Features of fractures of the anterior column of the acetabulum include:**

    a. disruption of the iliopubic line.
    b. medial displacement of the iliopubic column.
    c. medial displacement of the acetabular teardrop.
    d. disruption of the ilioischial line.
    e. anterior dislocation of the femoral head.

11. The following are true of fractures of the calcaneum:

a. Böhler's angle is normally 20–40 degrees.
b. it is the most commonly fractured tarsal bone.
c. most fractures do not involve the subtalar joint.
d. associated injuries are seen in 50%.
e. 10% are bilateral.

12. Following blunt abdominal trauma:

a. the spleen is the most frequently injured intraperitoneal organ.
b. the right lobe of the liver is more often injured than the left.
c. contrast-enhanced CT clearly demonstrates the site of pancreatic laceration in most cases.
d. bowel wall shows increased enhancement.
e. the gallbladder wall can appear focally thickened at US.

13. Signal-to-noise ratio in MRI is increased by:

a. increasing TE.
b. increasing the receive bandwidth.
c. increasing NEX.
d. reducing the number of phase encoding steps.
e. increasing voxel size.

14. Concerning the wrist:

a. the radiocarpal joint communicates with the midcarpal joint in up to 50%.
b. the flexor retinaculum attaches to the hook of the hamate.
c. flexor carpi ulnaris attaches to the pisiform.
d. the capitate normally articulates with the scaphoid.
e. the trapezoid is the last carpal bone to ossify.

15. With respect to imaging of the elbow:

a. most children with a visible posterior fat pad have a fracture.
b. CT is very useful for acute elbow trauma.
c. MRI should be performed with a surface coil.
d. the patients are best positioned prone in the MR scanner.
e. a lateral radiograph of the elbow is taken with the forearm supinated.

16. **Bone metastases:**

    a. can appear photopaenic at bone scintigraphy.
    b. occur to red marrow in over 90% of cases.
    c. when lytic, often involve the vertebral pedicles.
    d. from renal cell carcinoma are typically of high signal at T1-weighted MRI.
    e. from prostatic carcinoma often have a 'sunburst' periosteal reaction.

17. **Regarding osteosarcoma:**

    a. it most commonly occurs in patients aged over 40 years.
    b. the physis acts as a barrier to tumour spread.
    c. Paget's disease is a recognised risk factor.
    d. an aggressive periosteal reaction occurs.
    e. telangiectatic osteosarcoma usually has a lytic appearance.

18. **The following are true of intra-articular osteoid osteomas:**

    a. the knee is the commonest site.
    b. night pain is typical.
    c. plain radiographs show little reactive sclerosis.
    d. the 'double density' sign is often absent at bone scintigraphy.
    e. MRI is the investigation of choice.

19. **Giant cell tumours of bone:**

    a. are associated with Paget's disease.
    b. typically have a sclerotic margin.
    c. are confined by the periosteum.
    d. may contain low signal at T2-weighted MRI.
    e. are located centrally in the epiphysis.

20. **The arthropathy of systemic lupus erythematosus is associated with:**

    a. avascular necrosis of the femoral head.
    b. sclerosis of the terminal phalanges.
    c. erosions in most cases.
    d. Z-deformity of the thumb.
    e. plantar spurs.

21. With respect to the imaging features of the seronegative arthritides:

a. proliferative erosions occur in psoriatic arthropathy.
b. unilateral sacroiliac joint disease is common in ankylosing spondylitis.
c. symmetrical syndesmophytes are typical of Reiter's disease.
d. bone mineralization is usually normal in ankylosing spondylitis.
e. calcaneal new bone formation is a feature of psoriatic arthropathy.

22. Subchondral cysts occur in the following conditions:

a. osteoarthritis.
b. rheumatoid arthritis.
c. calcium pyrophosphate dihydrate deposition disease.
d. avascular necrosis.
e. sarcoid.

23. Hypertrophic osteoarthropathy:

a. is associated with mesothelioma.
b. usually extends onto the epiphyses.
c. shows increased uptake at bone scintigraphy.
d. produces a lamellar periosteal reaction.
e. is associated with hyperhidrosis.

24. The lateral third of the clavicle appears eroded in the following conditions:

a. rheumatoid arthritis.
b. ankylosing spondylitis.
c. hypoparathyroidism.
d. Langerhans' cell histiocytosis.
e. myeloma.

25. With respect to soft tissue calcification:

a. ligamentous calcification occurs in pseudoxanthoma elasticum.
b. tumoural calcinosis shows autosomal dominant inheritance.
c. calcific myonecrosis occurs 1–2 weeks after crush injury.
d. lesions in cysticercosis have a lucent centre.
e. calcification occurs in pseudopseudohypoparathyroidism.

26. Skeletal manifestations of sickle cell disease include:

a. osteopaenia and trabecular thinning.
b. 'fish' deformity of vertebrae.
c. 'bone-within-a-bone' appearance.
d. diffuse reduction in marrow signal at T1-weighted MRI.
e. avascular necrosis of the femoral head.

27. **The following are true of the skeletal manifestations of endocrine disease:**

  a. a short fourth metacarpal is a feature of hypothyroidism.
  b. fragmented epiphyses are seen in Turner's syndrome.
  c. hyperparathyroidism causes cortical tunnelling.
  d. joint spaces are widened in acromegaly.
  e. subperiosteal bone resorption is a sensitive indicator of hyperparathyroidism.

28. **Regarding multiple myeloma:**

  a. it is the commonest primary neoplasm of bone.
  b. generalised osteopaenia is a recognised appearance.
  c. scintigraphy overestimates disease extent.
  d. lesions can become sclerotic following chemotherapy.
  e. vertebral pedicle destruction is an early event.

29. **Desmoid tumours of bone:**

  a. are typically sclerotic.
  b. produce bony sequestrum.
  c. commonly metastasise.
  d. typically have ill-defined margins.
  e. invade the soft tissues.

30. **Aneurysmal bone cysts:**

  a. occur secondary to fibrous dysplasia.
  b. can present with scoliosis.
  c. may contain fluid–fluid levels at MR.
  d. do not contain matrix calcification.
  e. can cause the 'doughnut' sign at scintigraphy.

Module Two: Examination One – Answers

1. Answers

a. **True** – susceptibility artefact is less with FSE.
b. **False** – the amount of susceptibility artefact increases with B_0.
c. **False** – signal loss is greater at a longer TE.
d. **True**
e. **True** – the degree of distortion is inversely proportional to gradient strength.

(Guermazi A, Miaux Y, Zaim S et al. Metallic artefacts in MR imaging: effects of main field orientation and strength. *Clin Radiol* 2003;58:322–328)

2. Answers

a. **False** – medially.
b. **True**
c. **False** – the Achilles tendon does not have a tendon sheath.
d. **False** – inserts into fifth metatarsal, no muscles insert into the talus.
e. **True** – it is the unfused ossification centre of the posterior process of the talus.

(Butler et al. pp371–376)

3. Answers

a. **True**
b. **False** – coracoid process.
c. **True**
d. **False** – 5 cm for pelvis, 2.5 cm for both hips.
e. **False** – midway between the malleoli.

(Bell & Findlay pp96–135)

4. Answers

a. **True** – the nasal bones are usually fractured in isolation.
b. **True**
c. **True**
d. **False** – it involves both maxillary antra and extends across the midline above the hard palate.
e. **False** – LeFort I and II fractures are often associated with ZMC fractures, however.

(Harris & Harris pp63–97)

5. Answers

a. **True**
b. **True**
c. **False** – a single, obliquely-horizontal fracture line is typical.
d. **False** – the fragment arises from the anteroinferior corner.
e. **False** – it is stable.

(Harris & Harris pp199–203)

6. Answers

a. **True**
b. **True**
c. **False** – mid-third.
d. **False** – rare.
e. **False** – arterial injury is more common than venous.

(Rogers pp597–604)

7. Answers

a. **True**
b. **False** – > 80 degrees.
c. **False** – < 30 degrees.
d. **True**
e. **True** – 60% are associated with a scaphoid fracture at some time.

(Rogers pp855–861)

8. Answers

a. **True**
b. **False** – undisplaced.
c. **False** – lateral.
d. **True**
e. **True**

(Rogers pp1164–1169)

9. Answers

a. **False** – inferior and medial (inferolateral displacement suggests a haemarthrosis).
b. **False** – Hill–Sachs defects occur with a single dislocation in up to 70%.
c. **False** – this refers to a Bankart lesion.
d. **False** – Hill–Sachs defects are more commonly seen.
e. **False** – anterior dislocations account for 98%.

(Brant & Helms pp1011–1015)

10. Answers

a. **True**
b. **True**
c. **True**
d. **False** – this occurs with posterior rim fractures.
e. **False** – this is rare and is not a feature of anterior rim fracture.

(Rogers p989)

11. Answers

a. **True**
b. **True**
c. **False** – 75% involve the subtalar joint.
d. **True**
e. **True**

(Rogers pp1332–1333)

12. Answers

a. **True**
b. **True**
c. **False** – although pancreatic injury can be inferred, a fracture line is rarely visible.
d. **True** – due to delayed venous transit.
e. **True**

(Dähnert pp797–800)

13. Answers

a. **False** – allows more T2-dephasing to occur.
b. **False** – this increases the amount of noise.
c. **True**
d. **False** – reduces SNR.
e. **True**

(Hashemi & Bradley p169)

14. Answers

a. **True**
b. **True** – also to the pisiform, scaphoid tubercle and ridge of the trapezium.
c. **True**
d. **True**
e. **False** – the pisiform ossifies last.

(Butler et al. pp344–346)

15. Answers

a. **True** – approximately 80%.
b. **False** – limited value.
c. **True** – to improve SNR.
d. **True**
e. **False** – pronated.

(Rogers pp685–690)

16. Answers

a. **True** – when no blastic response occurs, or they outgrow their blood supply.
b. **True**
c. **True**
d. **False** – low signal due to fluid content.
e. **False** – this is rare, but is associated with prostatic carcinomas, retinoblastomas, neuroblastomas and GI tract malignancies.

(Brant & Helms p99; Dähnert pp117–119; Grainger & Allison pp1870–1872)

17. Answers

a. **False** – children and young adults.
b. **False**
c. **True** – 0.2–7.5% of patients with Paget's disease will develop osteosarcomas.
d. **True**
e. **True** – most telangiectatic osteosarcomas appear lytic, and may show aneurysmal expansion.

(Brant & Helms pp985–986; Dähnert pp138–141)

18. Answers

a. **False** – 13% of osteoid osteomas are intra-articular, most often in the hip.
b. **False** – unlike classical osteoid osteoma, night pain is not typical, and is often unresponsive to aspirin and NSAIDs.
c. **True** – little or no sclerosis is visible and the nidus is only seen in 28–50%.
d. **True** – generalised increased activity is seen within the joint instead.
e. **False** – CT is the preferred modality; MRI often fails to identify small niduses.

(Allen SA, Saifuddin A. Imaging of intra-articular osteoid osteomas. *Clin Radiol* 2003;58:845–852)

19. Answers

a. **True**
b. **False** – the margin is not sclerotic.
c. **False** – soft tissue extension occurs in up to 50%.
d. **True** – due to haemosiderin deposition.
e. **False** – eccentrically-located.

(Grainger & Allison pp1855–1858; Dähnert pp92–93)

20. Answers

a. **True**
b. **True** – also acro-osteolysis.
c. **False** – erosions are a rare feature of SLE arthropathy.
d. **True**
e. **False**

(Grainger & Allison pp2004–2005)

21. Answers

a. **True**
b. **False** – almost never occurs.
c. **False** – usually asymmetrical and non-marginal.
d. **True**
e. **True**

(Brant & Helms pp1028–1032)

22. Answers

a. **True**
b. **True**
c. **True**
d. **True**
e. **False**

(Brant & Helms pp1026–1027)

23. Answers

a. **True**
b. **False** – typically diametaphyseal.
c. **True**
d. **True**
e. **True**

(Grainger & Allison pp2024–2025; Dähnert pp103–104)

24. Answers

a. **True**
b. **False**
c. **False** – hyperparathyroidism is a cause, however.
d. **False**
e. **True**

(Chapman & Nakielny 2003 p51)

25. Answers

a. **True** – also dermal, vascular and tendinous calcification.
b. **True**
c. **False** – 1–2 months after injury.
d. **True**
e. **True**

(Grainger & Allison pp2079–2084)

26. Answers

a. **True**
b. **True**
c. **True**
d. **True**
e. **True**

(Grainger & Allison pp1904–1907; Dähnert pp158–159)

27. Answers

a. **False** – seen in Turner's syndrome, pseudohypoparathyroidism and pseudopseudohypoparathyroidism.
b. **False** – epiphyseal dysgenesis is a feature of hypothyroidism.
c. **True**
d. **True** – due to excess cartilage.
e. **False** – only seen in 10%.

(Grainger & Allison pp1939–1951)

28. Answers

a. **True**
b. **True** – in 15%.
c. **False** – underestimates extent.
d. **True** – also following radiotherapy.
e. **False**

(Grainger & Allison pp1913–1915; Dähnert pp121–122; Chapman & Nakielny 2003 pp575–576)

29. Answers

a. **False** – lytic.
b. **True**
c. **False** – do not metastasise.
d. **False** – well-defined as the lesion is slow growing.
e. **True**

(Brant & Helms pp991–992)

30. Answers

a. **True** – also to a variety of other bone tumours.
b. **True**
c. **True** – a non-specific finding.
d. **True**
e. **True** – this is a rim of increased activity.

(Grainger & Allison pp1854–1855; Dähnert p43)

Module Two: Examination Two – Questions

1. **Regarding weighting at spin echo MRI:**

   a. a long TR and a long TE result in T2-weighting.
   b. a short TR and a long TE results in proton density weighting.
   c. T1-weighting results from a TR of 500 ms and a TE of 15 ms.
   d. signal intensity depends only on the T1 and T2 of a tissue.
   e. T2*-weighted gradient echo uses the same TR and TE as T2-weighted spin echo sequences.

2. **Regarding the hip:**

   a. the capsule is strongest posteriorly.
   b. the capsule attaches proximal to the intertrochanteric line anteriorly.
   c. the femoral neck is anteverted by 15–20 degrees in the adult.
   d. the joint communicates with the psoas bursa.
   e. the ligamentum teres transmits blood vessels to the head of the femur.

3. **Concerning direct magnetic resonance arthrography:**

   a. epinephrine added to the gadolinium solution prolongs the duration of enhancement.
   b. an anterior approach to the shoulder is most common.
   c. gadolinium is not licensed for intra-articular use in the UK.
   d. injecting undiluted gadolinium results in very low signal at T1-weighted MRI.
   e. air bubbles can mimic loose bodies.

4. **Bone bruises detected at MRI:**

   a. are of low signal on gradient echo sequences using a low flip angle.
   b. enhance following IV Gd-DTPA.
   c. usually resolve within 3 months.
   d. are globular when due to an avulsion mechanism.
   e. are of high signal on STIR sequences.

5. **Concerning skull fractures:**

a. transverse fractures of the petrous temporal bone are more common than longitudinal.
b. CT can detect 0.5 ml of pneumocephalus.
c. 50–65% of linear skull fractures are demonstrable at axial CT.
d. diastatic sutural fractures are most common in the sagittal suture.
e. leptomeningeal cysts cause progressive widening of the fracture line.

6. **The Jefferson bursting fracture of C1:**

a. is due to axial loading in extension.
b. requires two fractures in each of the anterior and posterior arches.
c. results in a widened atlantodental interval on the open mouth view.
d. is associated with fractures of the occiput.
e. is best assessed using coronal reformats of helical CT data.

7. **The following are true concerning trauma to the proximal humerus:**

a. the greater tuberosity is seen in profile in external rotation.
b. the lesser tuberosity is seen in profile in internal rotation.
c. the commonest site for fracture is the anatomical neck.
d. isolated fractures of the anatomical neck are common.
e. avascular necrosis is a complication of fracture of the anatomical neck.

8. **Regarding injuries to the pelvis:**

a. violent contraction of sartorius can avulse the anterior inferior iliac spine.
b. isolated fractures of the iliac wing do not disrupt the pelvic ring.
c. Malgaigne pelvic ring disruption involves contralateral fractures of the pelvic ring.
d. the degree of pubic symphysis diastasis does not correlate with urethral injury.
e. insufficiency fractures of the pubic rami disrupt the pelvic ring at a single site.

9. **Regarding fractures of the femoral neck:**

a. most intertrochanteric fractures are comminuted.
b. avulsion of the greater trochanter usually occurs in adolescence.
c. avulsion of the lesser trochanter most frequently occurs in children.
d. isolated fractures of the femoral head are rare.
e. transverse subtrochanteric fractures are often pathological.

10. With respect to distal femoral fractures:

a. supracondylar fractures are often transverse.
b. extension into the knee joint is common with supracondylar fractures.
c. the distal fragment is usually anteriorly angulated.
d. they are associated with injury to the popliteal artery.
e. supracondylar fractures are associated with fracture-dislocation of the hip.

11. Regarding the menisci:

a. the lateral meniscus is more frequently torn than the medial.
b. anterior cruciate ligament tears are associated with tears of the lateral meniscus.
c. bucket handle tears are vertical longitudinal tears.
d. discoid menisci are more common medially.
e. discoid menisci are more prone to tears.

12. Regarding injury to the urinary tract:

a. most bladder ruptures are extraperitoneal.
b. intraperitoneal bladder rupture usually occurs at the dome.
c. ureteric injury is more common with blunt than penetrating trauma.
d. renal contusion causes a striated nephrogram at CT.
e. following renal artery avulsion, rim enhancement of the kidney can occur.

13. Multi-slice CT:

a. uses third generation beam-detector geometry.
b. requires all the detectors to have the same width in the z-axis.
c. permits isotropic voxel dimensions.
d. uses a cone beam of x-rays.
e. uses the same reconstruction algorithms as helical CT.

14. The following are true of the normal shoulder joint:

a. the glenohumeral ligaments lie posteriorly.
b. the subacromial bursa communicates with the joint.
c. teres minor attaches to the lesser tuberosity of the humerus.
d. the glenoid labrum is deficient inferiorly.
e. the tendon of the long head of biceps is extrasynovial.

15. **Regarding knee arthrography:**

a. no patient preparation is required.
b. meniscal cysts are better seen on delayed films.
c. 10 ml of air is sufficient for double-contrast.
d. anaphylactoid reactions can occur to intra-articular iodinated contrast.
e. patients are examined in the prone position.

16. **Bone metastases from the following primary tumours are usually sclerotic:**

a. prostate.
b. lung.
c. bladder.
d. breast.
e. bronchial carcinoid.

17. **Chondrocalcinosis is associated with:**

a. haemochromatosis.
b. untreated hyperparathyroidism.
c. gout.
d. ochronosis.
e. synovial osteochondromatosis.

18. **Concerning malignant lesions of bone:**

a. chordoma is most common in the thoracolumbar spine.
b. fibrosarcoma is the commonest tumour secondary to Paget's disease.
c. adamantinoma occurs in the tibia in over 90% of cases.
d. angiosarcoma has a 'soap bubble' appearance at radiography.
e. periosteal osteosarcoma is often seen to invade the medullary cavity at MRI.

19. **Osteochondromas:**

a. are usually painful.
b. are commonly found in the metaphysis of long bones.
c. cause metaphyseal widening.
d. which grow after epiphyseal fusion are suggestive of malignant transformation.
e. are confined to the cortex.

20. **Simple bone cysts:**
    a. are unilocular by definition.
    b. are most common in the calcaneus.
    c. elicit a florid periosteal reaction.
    d. are definitively treated by curettage.
    e. can demonstrate a 'fallen fragment' sign without fracture.

21. **Regarding gout:**
    a. joint space is preserved until late in the disease.
    b. bone mineralization is usually normal.
    c. tophi are of low signal at T1-weighted MRI.
    d. radiographic changes often predate the first attack.
    e. erosions characteristically have overhanging margins.

22. **Regarding osteoarthritis:**
    a. articular cartilage returns increased signal at T2-weighted MRI.
    b. knee involvement is most common in the patellofemoral compartment.
    c. new bone formation occurs at the lateral margin of the femoral neck.
    d. geodes are pathognomonic.
    e. the femoral head commonly migrates medially.

23. **Pseudofractures occur in:**
    a. Paget's disease.
    b. fibrous dysplasia.
    c. long-term treatment with phenytoin.
    d. scurvy.
    e. osteogenesis imperfecta.

24. **Concerning sarcoid:**
    a. the long bones are preferentially affected.
    b. joint involvement is common.
    c. a lace-like trabecular pattern of bone destruction is seen.
    d. osteosclerotic changes are typical in the skull.
    e. vertebral involvement is common.

25. **Dense metaphyseal bands are seen in the following conditions:**
    a. treated rickets.
    b. thyroid acropachy.
    c. hypervitaminosis A.
    d. scurvy.
    e. lead poisoning.

26. **Regarding the triangular fibrocartilage complex:**

a. peripheral tears can heal spontaneously.
b. perforation is more common with positive ulnar variance.
c. tears are best demonstrated at axial MRI.
d. intrasubstance degeneration is best seen at proton density MRI.
e. a biconcave appearance at coronal MRI is abnormal.

27. **The following are causes of diffuse osteosclerosis:**

a. myelofibrosis.
b. osteopetrosis.
c. sickle cell disease.
d. fluorosis.
e. achondroplasia.

28. **Regarding tuberculosis of bone:**

a. osteomyelitis is more common in adults than children.
b. osteomyelitis usually presents as a poorly-defined lytic lesion.
c. the hip and knee joints are common sites of tuberculous arthritis.
d. spondylitis preferentially affects the posterior vertebral elements.
e. diffuse sclerosis of bone is the commonest pattern.

29. **Diffuse idiopathic skeletal hyperostosis:**

a. is associated with HLA-B27 in 60–70%.
b. is more common on the right side of the thoracic spine.
c. is associated with sacroiliitis.
d. is associated with ossification of the patellar ligament.
e. is asymptomatic.

30. **Neuropathic osteoarthropathy:**

a. due to syringomyelia is usually confined to the upper limb.
b. is most often of the hypertrophic form.
c. causes phalangeal tapering.
d. is a cause of loose bodies.
e. is characteristically associated with minimal joint effusion.

Module Two: Examination Two – Answers

1. Answers

a. **True**
b. **False** – proton density uses long TR and a short TE.
c. **True**
d. **False** – it also depends on the number of mobile protons in a voxel.
e. **False** – gradient echo uses much shorter timing parameters.

(Hashemi & Bradley pp49–55)

2. Answers

a. **False** – strongest anteriorly, reinforced by the iliofemoral ligament.
b. **False** – attaches along the intertrochanteric crest.
c. **False** – 8 degrees.
d. **True**
e. **True** – although this is relatively unimportant in adults.

(Butler et al. pp357–360)

3. Answers

a. **True** – e.g. 0.3 ml of 1:1000 epinephrine for a shoulder.
b. **True** – although the posterior approach is becoming more common.
c. **False** – it has been licensed since January 2004.
d. **True** – also at T2-weighting.
e. **True** – although they are usually found in the non-dependent parts of the joint.

(Grainger AJ, Elliott JM, Campbell RSD et al. Direct MR arthrography: a review of current use. *Clin Radiol* 2000;55:163–176)

4. Answers

a. **False** – high signal – a low flip angle is used for T2-weighting.
b. **True** – although enhancement is minimal, and often delayed.
c. **True** – symptoms typically last six weeks.
d. **False** – such bruises are linear and perpendicular to the axis of avulsion.
e. **True**

(Eustace S, Keogh C, Blake RJ et al. MR imaging of bone oedema: mechanisms and interpretation. *Clin Radiol* 2001;56:4–12)

5. Answers

a. **False** – longitudinal fractures are more common.
b. **True**
c. **False** – only 20% are seen.
d. **False** – the lambdoid and coronal sutures are the commonest sites.
e. **True** – this usually occurs following injury at a young age.

(Harris & Harris pp1–14)

6. Answers

a. **False** – it requires axial loading with the neck in a neutral position.
b. **False** – a single anterior and single posterior fracture is sufficient.
c. **True**
d. **True** – occipital condyle fractures may occur.
e. **False** – axial views are optimal.

(Harris & Harris pp251–253)

7. Answers

a. **True**
b. **True**
c. **False** – surgical neck.
d. **False** – unusual.
e. **True**

(Rogers pp632–637)

8. Answers

a. **False** – sartorius avulses the anterior superior iliac spine.
b. **True**
c. **False** – the fractures are ipsilateral.
d. **True**
e. **True**

(Harris & Harris pp732–776)

9. Answers

a. **True**
b. **False** – elderly patients most often.
c. **True**
d. **True**
e. **True**

(Rogers pp1058–1069)

10. Answers

a. **True** – or slightly obliquely orientated.
b. **True**
c. **False** – posteriorly angulated.
d. **True**
e. **True**

(Rogers p1134)

11. Answers

a. **False** – the commonest site is the posterior horn of the medial meniscus.
b. **True**
c. **True**
d. **False** – laterally, in approximately 3% of the population.
e. **True**

(Brant & Helms pp1083–1087)

12. Answers

a. **True** – 80–90%.
b. **True** – extraperitoneal rupture is most common around the bladder neck.
c. **False** – penetrating trauma is more common.
d. **True**
e. **True** – due to collaterals.

(Wah TM, Spencer JA. The role of CT in the management of adult urinary tract trauma. *Clin Radiol* 2001;56:268–277)

13. Answers

a. **True**
b. **False** – some systems use matrix arrays of detectors with the same z-axis width, others have adaptive arrays where detector width increases peripherally.
c. **True**
d. **True**
e. **False** – the 180 and 360 degree interpolation algorithms used for helical CT are inadequate for multi-slice CT.

(Dawson P, Lees WR. Multi-slice technology in computed tomography. *Clin Radiol* 2001;56:302–309)

14. Answers

a. **False** – anteriorly.
b. **False** – communication indicates rupture of supraspinatus.
c. **False** – the inferior facet of the greater tuberosity.
d. **False** – it is a complete ring, unlike the acetabular labrum.
e. **True** – but intracapsular.

(Butler et al. pp335–336)

15. Answers

a. **True**
b. **True**
c. **False** – 40 ml.
d. **True**
e. **True**

(Chapman & Nakielny 2001 pp265–268)

16. Answers

a. **True**
b. **False**
c. **False**
d. **False**
e. **True**

(Grainger & Allison pp1872–1874; Chapman & Nakielny 2003 p18)

17. Answers

a. **True**
b. **True**
c. **True**
d. **True**
e. **False**

(Brant & Helms pp1034–1036)

18. Answers

a. **False** – 85–90% occur in the basisphenoid and sacrum.
b. **False** – osteosarcoma in 50%, fibrosarcoma/malignant fibrous histiocytoma in 25%.
c. **True**
d. **True**
e. **False** – no cortical or medullary invasion occurs.

(Grainger & Allison pp1886–1887 & pp1895–1896)

19. Answers

a. **False** – usually asymptomatic, but can be painful with impingement of nerves or vessels.
b. **True**
c. **True**
d. **True** – suggestive of degeneration into chondrosarcoma or osteosarcoma.
e. **False** – in continuity with the marrow and cortex.

(Dähnert pp131–132)

20. Answers

a. **False** – they are not always unilocular.
b. **False** – 80% occur in the proximal humerus and femur.
c. **False** – no periosteal reaction in the absence of a fracture.
d. **False** – there is a 50% recurrence after curettage.
e. **False** – the fallen fragment sign is only seen once a fracture has occurred.

(Grainger & Allison pp1852–1854)

21. Answers

a. **True**
b. **True**
c. **False** – tophi are isointense to muscle at T1-weighting, and low signal at T2.
d. **False** – radiographic changes do not occur for 5–10 years after the index episode.
e. **True**

(Grainger & Allison pp2012–2013; Dähnert pp94–96)

22. Answers

a. **True**
b. **False** – mainly medial tibiofemoral compartment.
c. **False** – buttressing occurs medially.
d. **False** – seen in a variety of conditions.
e. **False** – usually superolaterally.

(Grainger & Allison pp2016–2017; Dähnert p129)

23. Answers

a. **True**
b. **True**
c. **True** – phenytoin can cause osteomalacia.
d. **False**
e. **True**

(Dähnert p145)

24. Answers

a. **False** – small bones of hands and feet.
b. **False** – it is rare.
c. **True**
d. **False** – usually osteolytic.
e. **False** – rare.

(Brant & Helms p1037; Dähnert p157)

25. Answers

a. **True**
b. **False**
c. **False** – hypervitaminosis D.
d. **True** – the 'white line of Frankl'.
e. **True** – also phosphorus and bismuth poisoning.

(Grainger & Allison p1963)

26. Answers

a. **True** – the periphery is vascularised, unlike the central TFCC.
b. **True**
c. **False** – coronal MRI.
d. **False** – T2*-weighted gradient echo sequences are superior.
e. **False** – this is the normal appearance.

(Grainger & Allison p2049)

27. Answers

a. **True**
b. **True**
c. **True**
d. **True**
e. **False**

(Brant & Helms pp1054–1057)

28. Answers

a. **False** – osteomyelitis is more common in children, especially under 5 years.
b. **True**
c. **True**
d. **False** – vertebral body.
e. **False**

(Brant & Helms p250; Dähnert pp169–170)

29. Answers

a. **False** – HLA-B27 positive in 30%.
b. **True** – due to aortic pulsation on the left.
c. **False**
d. **True** – also of the iliolumbar, sacroiliac, sacrotuberous, coracoclavicular and posterior longitudinal ligaments.
e. **False** – back pain may occur.

(Grainger & Allison p2020; Dähnert pp66–67)

30. Answers

a. **True**
b. **False** – the atrophic form is most common.
c. **True** – secondary to concentric atrophy.
d. **True**
e. **False** – effusions are usually large and persistent.

(Grainger & Allison p2019; Dähnert pp125–126)

Module Two: Examination Three – Questions

1. **Concerning artefacts in MRI:**

   a. aliasing occurs in the frequency-encoding direction.
   b. chemical shift artefact is reduced by a higher field strength magnet.
   c. crosstalk is reduced by increasing the interslice gap.
   d. magic angle artefact occurs when a tendon lies at 55 degrees to the phase encoding gradient.
   e. motion artefact is seen in the direction of phase encoding.

2. **An axial MRI through the tibiofemoral compartment of the knee joint shows the following:**

   a. the anterior cruciate crossing medially to the posterior cruciate ligament.
   b. the lateral head of gastrocnemius.
   c. popliteus.
   d. the medial collateral ligament.
   e. vastus intermedius.

3. **Regarding isotope bone scintigraphy:**

   a. corticosteroid therapy increases bone uptake of tracer.
   b. ^{99m}Tc-MDP is excreted by glomerular filtration.
   c. the effective dose is approximately 7–10 mSv.
   d. increased activity is seen in skull sutures.
   e. three phase studies are an integral part of routine examinations.

4. **Features of a blow-out fracture of the orbit include:**

   a. limitation of down gaze.
   b. an intact inferior orbital rim.
   c. a soft tissue mass in the superior maxillary antrum.
   d. orbital emphysema.
   e. an air–fluid level in the frontal sinus.

5. **Regarding mandibular injuries:**

   a. the coronoid process is the commonest site of fracture.
   b. the mandible is most often fractured in a single site only.
   c. with the mouth open, the mandibular condyle may normally sublux.
   d. there is an association with haemotympanum.
   e. bilateral parasymphyseal fractures result in obstruction of the oral airway.

6. **Concerning dens fractures:**

   a. avulsion of the tip is a type I fracture.
   b. type I fractures are the commonest injury of C2.
   c. type II fractures have a low incidence of non-union.
   d. type III fractures disrupt the axis 'ring of Harris' on the lateral radiograph.
   e. non-union of a type III fracture results in an os odontoideum.

7. **The following are true of scapular injuries:**

   a. road traffic accidents are the commonest cause.
   b. other injuries are present in 20–40%.
   c. acromial fractures are usually vertically orientated.
   d. coracoid fractures are usually vertically orientated.
   e. glenoid fractures are best seen in oblique projections.

8. **Regarding fractures of the olecranon and proximal ulna:**

   a. most fractures are obliquely orientated.
   b. a posterior fat pad is visible at radiography.
   c. isolated fracture of the coronoid process is unusual.
   d. the olecranon apophysis can be mistaken for a fracture.
   e. fracture through the anterior trochlear notch is associated with posterior dislocation.

9. **Concerning ligamentous injuries of the knee:**

   a. posterior cruciate ligament tears are usually an isolated injury.
   b. medial collateral ligament tears are best assessed at coronal MRI.
   c. lateral collateral ligament injuries are usually due to a varus force.
   d. sprains appear as increased signal at T1-weighted MRI.
   e. the anterior cruciate ligament is best seen at sagittal oblique MRI.

10. **Regarding stress and insufficiency fractures of the neck of femur:**

   a. insufficiency fractures are usually subcapital.
   b. stress fractures are most often transcervical.
   c. stress fractures are of low intensity at T1-weighted MRI.
   d. stress fractures extend to a cortex at MRI imaging.
   e. stress fractures have surrounding high signal at T2-weighted MRI.

11. Lisfranc injuries:

a. are often purely ligamentous.
b. are associated with diabetes mellitus.
c. are more often divergent than homolateral.
d. are associated with cuboid fractures.
e. are most common at the 2nd to 4th metatarsals.

12. Concerning traumatic rupture of the diaphragm:

a. it is most often left-sided.
b. a defect of less than 10 mm is treated conservatively.
c. chest radiography is non-diagnostic in 20–30%.
d. it is best diagnosed with T2*-weighted sagittal MRI.
e. delayed radiographs at 6 hours are useful if the initial chest film is equivocal.

13. The acquisition time of an MRI study depends directly on the following:

a. TR.
b. TE.
c. the number of phase-encoding steps.
d. TI.
e. field of view in the frequency-encoding direction.

14. With respect to the anatomy of the elbow:

a. the medial condyle is more prominent than the lateral.
b. the extensor muscles of the forearm arise from the medial condyle.
c. the brachialis muscle inserts at the coronoid process.
d. the radial head articulates with the capitellum.
e. the annular ligament encircles the radial head.

15. Concerning radiography of the knee:

a. the foot is internally rotated by 10 degrees for an AP view.
b. the anterior intercondylar notch is shown by angling the central ray by 110 degrees.
c. the patient is supine for a skyline view of the patella.
d. the leg is rotated medially for an oblique view of the tibiofibular joint.
e. the knee is fully extended for a horizontal beam lateral.

16. **Parosteal osteosarcoma:**

a. is more common than periosteal osteosarcoma.
b. is more common in older patients than conventional osteosarcoma.
c. arises at the distal femur in most cases.
d. is commonly separated from normal bone by a radiolucent line.
e. has a worse prognosis than telangiectatic osteosarcoma.

17. **Primary lymphoma of bone:**

a. is most often Hodgkin's lymphoma.
b. is most common in the skull and vertebral column.
c. elicits reactive bone sclerosis in up to half of cases.
d. usually has a soft tissue mass at presentation.
e. responds poorly to radiotherapy.

18. **Non-ossifying fibromas:**

a. are extremely painful.
b. interrupt the bone cortex at CT.
c. are commonly seen around the knee.
d. demonstrate increased uptake at bone scintigraphy.
e. are associated with café au lait spots.

19. **Chondroblastomas:**

a. are typically found in the diaphysis.
b. mainly occur in patients under 30 years.
c. are asymptomatic in most cases.
d. elicit a periosteal reaction.
e. are associated with solitary bone cysts.

20. **Erosive osteoarthritis shows a predilection for the following joints:**

a. sacroiliac.
b. shoulder.
c. acromioclavicular.
d. temporomandibular.
e. symphysis pubis.

21. **Regarding diseases which affect joints:**

a. patchy osteoporosis is a feature of reflex sympathetic dystrophy.
b. sarcoid typically affects the shoulders and elbows.
c. pigmented villonodular synovitis causes high signal within the joint space at T2-weighted MRI.
d. epiphyseal enlargement is a feature of haemophilia A.
e. sharply demarcated erosions occur in multicentric reticulocytosis.

22. Concerning synovial chondromatosis:

a. it is most common in the knee joint.
b. joint effusions are a common feature.
c. joint locking occurs.
d. MRI shows nodules attached to the synovium by a pedicle.
e. there is no malignant potential.

23. Regarding avascular necrosis:

a. subchondral lucency is a consistent feature of early disease.
b. it results in collapse and fragmentation of the articular surface.
c. aspirin is a recognised cause.
d. CT is more sensitive than MRI in making the diagnosis.
e. most cases in the UK are due to chronic corticosteroid use.

24. Skeletal manifestations of Cushing's syndrome include:

a. biconcave vertebral bodies.
b. depression of callus formation.
c. reduced osteophyte formation.
d. enthesopathy.
e. insufficiency fractures.

25. Lesions containing a fluid–fluid level at MRI include:

a. giant cell tumour.
b. fibrous dysplasia.
c. enchondroma.
d. simple bone cyst.
e. malignant fibrous histiocytoma.

26. A divergent, spiculated ('sunray') periosteal reaction occurs with:

a. tuberculosis.
b. syphilis.
c. osteosarcoma.
d. fibrous dysplasia.
e. tropical ulcer.

27. With regards to the detection of soft tissue foreign bodies with US:

a. smooth-surfaced bodies usually cast clean acoustic shadows.
b. glass often demonstrates reverberation artefacts.
c. an inflammatory reaction aids detection.
d. a stand-off pad is routinely necessary.
e. US has a sensitivity in excess of 90%.

28. **Concerning MRI of skeletal muscle:**

   a. normal muscle is of lower signal intensity than fat on STIR sequences.
   b. in polymyositis, muscle oedema is most marked in vastus lateralis.
   c. subacute denervation causes muscle oedema.
   d. corticosteroid use causes fatty infiltration.
   e. myositis ossificans results in foci of low signal with a high signal rim at T1-weighting.

29. **The following are features of Gaucher's disease:**

   a. subarticular lucency in the femoral head.
   b. endosteal scalloping.
   c. increased incidence of osteomyelitis.
   d. notching of the superior rib border.
   e. splenomegaly in adult-onset disease.

30. **Features of renal osteodystrophy include:**

   a. elevated serum parathyroid hormone.
   b. a 'superscan' at bone scintigraphy.
   c. bone resorption most marked on the sacral side of the sacroiliac joint.
   d. osteosclerosis, which increases following renal transplantation.
   e. periarticular calcification.

Module Two: Examination Three – Answers

1. Answers

a. **True**
b. **False** – this increases the difference in precessional frequency between fat and water protons.
c. **True**
d. **False** – occurs when tendons are 55 degrees to the main field, B_0.
e. **True**

(Hashemi & Bradley pp175–186)

2. Answers

a. **False** – the ACL passes laterally to the PCL.
b. **True**
c. **True**
d. **True**
e. **False**

(Butler et al. pp363–367)

3. Answers

a. **False** – reduces uptake.
b. **True**
c. **False** – 3.8 mSv.
d. **True**
e. **False** – performed when bone tumours or primary infection is suspected.

(Brant & Helms pp1227–1231)

4. Answers

a. **False** – limitation of upwards and outward gaze.
b. **True** – the floor of the orbit is fractured, but the inferior orbital rim is intact.
c. **True**
d. **True**
e. **False**

(Harris & Harris pp66–72)

5. Answers

a. **False** – most fractures occur in the body, in the region of the mandibular foramen.
b. **True** – though multiple fractures are not uncommon.
c. **True**
d. **True** – due to fractures of the external auditory meatus.
e. **True** – due to retraction of the detached symphysis and tongue.

(Harris & Harris pp111–118)

6. Answers

a. **True**
b. **False** – type II fractures, through the base of the dens, are the most common.
c. **False** – non-union occurs in 30–50%.
d. **True** – this may be the only sign on a lateral film.
e. **False** – type II fractures lead to os odontoideum.

(Harris & Harris pp239–243)

7. Answers

a. **True**
b. **False** – 80%.
c. **True**
d. **False** – transversely orientated.
e. **True**

(Rogers pp619–632)

8. Answers

a. **False** – transverse.
b. **True**
c. **True**
d. **True**
e. **False** – anterior.

(Rogers pp705–708)

9. Answers

a. **False** – they are isolated in only 30%.
b. **True**
c. **True**
d. **True**
e. **True**

(Haaga et al. pp1880–1887; Dähnert p60)

10. Answers

a. **True**
b. **False** – basicervical.
c. **True**
d. **True**
e. **True**

(Rogers pp1053–1054)

11. Answers

a. **False** – the injury usually involves metatarsal fractures.
b. **True**
c. **False** – homolateral Lisfranc injuries are more common.
d. **True**
e. **True**

(Harris & Harris p882–887)

12. Answers

a. **True** – 72–88% in clinical series.
b. **False** – surgery is mandatory.
c. **False** – it is non-diagnostic in over half of cases.
d. **False** – T1-weighted MRI is the preferred means of assessment.
e. **True**

(Grainger & Allison p538)

13. Answers

a. **True** – for a spin echo study, acquisition time = TR × NEX × $N_{phase\ encoding}$.
b. **False**
c. **True**
d. **False**
e. **False**

(Hashemi & Bradley pp167–173)

14. Answers

a. **True**
b. **False** – lateral.
c. **True**
d. **True**
e. **True**

(Rogers pp683–685)

15. Answers

a. **False** – the leg is not rotated.
b. **True** – 90 degrees for the posterior intercondylar notch.
c. **False** – prone, with the knee flexed 90 degrees.
d. **True**
e. **False** – flexed 20–30 degrees.

(Bell & Findlay pp106–110)

16. Answers

a. **True** – it accounts for 5% of all osteosarcomas.
b. **True** – 50% are over 30 years, versus 25% of central osteosarcomas.
c. **True** – it occurs at the posterior femoral metaphysis in 50–60%.
d. **False** – seen in 30–40%, this is not a feature of periosteal osteosarcoma.
e. **False** – it has the best prognosis of all forms of osteosarcoma.

(Grainger & Allison pp1885–1886; Dähnert p140)

17. Answers

a. **False** – usually B-cell non-Hodgkin's lymphoma.
b. **False** – most common in the diaphyses of long bones, and the pelvis.
c. **True**
d. **False** – there is no soft tissue mass in 50%.
e. **False**

(Grainger & Allison pp1892–1894)

18. Answers

a. **False** – painless.
b. **True** – due to cortical replacement by benign fibrous tissue.
c. **True**
d. **True**
e. **True** – associated with neurofibromatosis.

(Brant & Helms pp969–971)

19. Answers

a. **False** – they are epiphyseal lesions.
b. **True**
c. **False** – chrondroblastomas most often present with pain.
d. **True** – a linear periosteal reaction occurs in one third.
e. **False** – aneurysmal bone cysts may develop, however.

(Grainger & Allison pp1843–1844)

20. Answers

a. **True**
b. **False**
c. **True**
d. **True**
e. **True**

(Brant & Helms pp1026–1027)

21. Answers

a. **True**
b. **False** – hands.
c. **False** – typically low signal.
d. **True**
e. **True**

(Brant & Helms pp1035–1041)

22. Answers

a. **True** – accounts for over half of cases.
b. **False** – effusions are uncommon.
c. **True** – due to loose bodies.
d. **True** – nodules are initially tethered to the synovium.
e. **False** – dedifferentiation into chondrosarcoma may occur.

(Grainger & Allison pp2020–2021; Dähnert pp162–163)

23. Answers

a. **False** – a late and unreliable sign.
b. **True**
c. **True**
d. **False** – MRI is more sensitive.
e. **False** – most cases are idiopathic.

(Brant & Helms pp1073–1074)

24. Answers

- a. **True**
- b. **False** – exuberant callus formation, resulting in marginal condensation of wedged vertebrae.
- c. **True**
- d. **False**
- e. **True**

(Grainger & Allison pp1930–1931)

25. Answers

- a. **True**
- b. **True**
- c. **False**
- d. **True**
- e. **True**

(Chapman & Nakielny 2003 p62)

26. Answers

- a. **True**
- b. **True** – also a parallel spiculated, 'hair on end' reaction.
- c. **True**
- d. **False** – no periosteal reaction in the absence of fracture.
- e. **True**

(Chapman & Nakielny 2003 p34)

27. Answers

- a. **False** – smooth and flat bodies usually cast 'dirty' shadows, bodies with an irregular surface or small radius of curvature cast 'clean' shadows.
- b. **True** – as does metal.
- c. **True** – by producing a rim of low reflectivity around the foreign body.
- d. **False** – the near-field resolution of a modern transducer is sufficient.
- e. **True** – 95%.

(Boyse TD, Fessell DP, Jacobson JA et al. Ultrasound of soft tissue foreign bodies and associated complications with surgical correlation. *Radiographics* 2001;21:1251–1256)

28. Answers

- a. **False** – fat is of lower signal than muscle.
- b. **True** – also vastus medialis, with relative sparing of biceps femoris and rectus femoris.
- c. **True**
- d. **True**
- e. **False** – high signal centre (fat) surrounded by signal void (calcification).

(May DA, Disler DG, Jones EA et al. Abnormal signal intensity in skeletal muscle at MR imaging: patterns, pearls and pitfalls. *Radiographics* 2000;20:S295–S315)

29. Answers

a. **True** – due to avascular necrosis.
b. **True**
c. **True**
d. **False**
e. **True**

(Grainger & Allison pp1918–1920; Dähnert pp91–92)

30. Answers

a. **True** – in up to two-thirds.
b. **True**
c. **False** – subchondral bone resorption is most marked on the iliac side.
d. **True** – osteosclerosis can also decrease following transplantation.
e. **True**

(Grainger & Allison pp1935–1938; Dähnert pp149–150)

MODULE THREE

Gastrointestinal and Hepatobiliary

Time Allowed: 2 hours

Module Three: Examination One – Questions

1. **Hyoscine N-butylbromide:**

   a. has an immediate onset of action following IV injection.
   b. has no effect on the lower oesophageal sphincter.
   c. reduces small bowel transit time.
   d. is contraindicated in myasthenia gravis.
   e. has a 15-minute duration of action.

2. **Regarding suspensions of barium sulphate used in gastrointestinal radiology:**

   a. the barium particles are 0.1–5 mm in diameter.
   b. suspensions are non-ionic.
   c. suspensions are of alkaline pH.
   d. simethicone acts as an anti-flocculation agent.
   e. mucosal detail is improved by heterogeneous particle size.

3. **Contraindications to double-contrast barium enema include:**

   a. pseudomembranous colitis.
   b. rectal biopsy at flexible sigmoidoscopy 48 hours previously.
   c. toxic megacolon.
   d. rectovaginal fistula.
   e. suspected perforation.

4. **Regarding the peritoneal spaces:**

   a. the left paracolic gutter communicates with the left subphrenic space.
   b. the right infracolic space is larger than the left.
   c. the superior recess of the lesser sac surrounds the quadrate lobe of the liver.
   d. up to 100 ml of peritoneal fluid is normal.
   e. the right and left subphrenic spaces do not communicate directly.

5. **The duodenum:**

   a. takes its blood supply from a branch of the superior mesenteric artery.
   b. is shortest in its third part.
   c. is posterior to the common bile duct in its second part.
   d. is crossed anteriorly by the superior mesenteric vein.
   e. has the ampulla of Vater at the anteromedial wall of the second part.

6. **Concerning the salivary glands:**
   a. the parotid duct opens opposite the second upper molar.
   b. the parotid is of higher attenuation than skeletal muscle at unenhanced CT.
   c. the submandibular gland is of higher attenuation than the parotid at unenhanced CT.
   d. the sublingual gland has a 7 cm long duct at sialography.
   e. accessory parotid tissue is present in 15–25% of people.

7. **The speed of sound:**
   a. is inversely proportional to the bulk modulus of elasticity of a medium.
   b. is proportional to the density of a medium.
   c. is independent of the acoustic intensity of the beam.
   d. is greater in fat than in liver.
   e. is assumed to be constant by the US machine.

8. **Concerning the resolution of a real-time grey-scale US image:**
   a. axial resolution is approximately half the length of the transmitted pulse.
   b. axial resolution is independent of transmit frequency.
   c. lateral resolution is dependent on beam width.
   d. contrast resolution depends on the width of the beam in the elevation plane.
   e. temporal resolution is independent of the width of the field of view.

9. **Regarding salivary gland tumours:**
   a. they are more common in the parotid than the submandibular gland.
   b. pleomorphic adenoma is of low signal at T2-weighted MRI.
   c. adenoid cystic carcinoma most often arises in the submandibular gland.
   d. parotid adenolymphoma appears well-circumscribed at US.
   e. mucoepidermoid carcinoma contains cystic areas at CT.

10. **Regarding achalasia:**
   a. there is an association with oesophageal carcinoma.
   b. 'beaking' of the gastro-oesophageal junction is best demonstrated on a prone barium swallow.
   c. hot fluids exacerbate the symptoms.
   d. surgery is more effective than pneumatic dilatation of the gastro-oesophageal junction.
   e. the diagnosis can be established by scintigraphy.

11. **Oesophageal leiomyomas:**

a. cause filling defects with an obtuse angle to the adjacent mucosa.
b. are most common in the middle third of the oesophagus.
c. are commonly multiple.
d. rarely calcify.
e. are rarely symptomatic.

12. **Concerning oesophageal carcinoma:**

a. squamous cell carcinoma is the commonest form.
b. squamous cell carcinoma is associated with coeliac disease.
c. alcohol misuse is a risk factor.
d. contact with the aorta over less than 90 degrees suggests a potentially resectable lesion.
e. lesions are usually of increased reflectivity at EUS.

13. **Concerning the radiology of the post-operative stomach:**

a. post-operative ulcers are more common in the efferent loop of a gastrojejunostomy.
b. recurrent ulcers in the gastric remnant are common.
c. outlet obstruction due to submucosal haemorrhage is commonly self-limiting.
d. efferent loop obstruction is usually due to herniation behind the anastomosis.
e. jejunogastric intussusception most often involves the efferent loop.

14. **Menetrier's disease:**

a. is associated with gastric gland atrophy.
b. causes focal fold enlargement most marked on the lesser curve.
c. characteristically produces enlarged, stiffened gastric folds.
d. involves the antrum in 70–80% of cases.
e. causes increased fluid in the small bowel at CT.

15. **At a double-contrast barium meal, a gastric ulcer is more likely to be benign if the following findings are present:**

a. Hampton's line.
b. extension beyond the gastric wall.
c. a Carman meniscus.
d. nodular gastric folds.
e. a linear shape to the ulcer.

16. **Regarding stent insertion for gastric and duodenal strictures:**

a. uncovered stents are preferred.
b. a nasogastric tube is required, to insufflate the stomach with CO_2.
c. use of hydrophilic guidewires is associated with increased risk of tumour perforation.
d. post-deployment balloon dilatation is not usually required.
e. the technical success rate is significantly less than for oesophageal strictures.

17. **Regarding radiological percutaneous gastrostomy:**

a. ascites is an absolute contraindication.
b. it is not suitable for patients who have undergone partial gastrectomy.
c. the catheter should be directed towards the pylorus.
d. major complications are less frequent than with percutaneous endoscopic gastrostomy.
e. peri-catheter leakage is common in peritoneal dialysis patients.

18. **Regarding the imaging of malignant gastrointestinal stromal tumours:**

a. they are well-circumscribed at CT.
b. peritoneal lymphadenopathy is common.
c. bone metastases are present in a minority.
d. ascites is rare.
e. a desmoplastic response in the mesentery is common.

19. **The following are features of mastocytosis:**

a. angioneurotic oedema.
b. thickened valvulae conniventes.
c. mucosal nodules more common in the distal small bowel.
d. gastrointestinal haemorrhage.
e. mesenteric lymphadenopathy.

20. **CT findings in tuberculous peritonitis include:**

a. mesenteric lymphadenopathy.
b. nodular thickening of the peritoneum.
c. low attenuation (0–10 HU) ascites.
d. loculation of fluid collections.
e. scalloping of the liver edge.

21. Concerning the intestinal polyposis syndromes:

a. epidermoid cysts occur in Turcot's syndrome.
b. intestinal hamartomas are a feature of Cowden's syndrome.
c. abdominal wall desmoids occur in familial adenomatous polyposis.
d. keratoacanthomas occur in Cronkhite–Canada syndrome.
e. in Peutz–Jeghers syndrome, the risk of thyroid carcinoma is increased.

22. Regarding CT colonography:

a. it is superior to barium enema in detecting colorectal adenomas.
b. polyethylene glycol is preferable to phosphosoda bowel preparation.
c. extracolonic findings requiring further assessment are detected in 10%.
d. supine positioning improves sigmoid distension.
e. a shift in position between prone and supine datasets reliably distinguishes faecal residue from a polyp.

23. Colonic angiodysplasia:

a. is most common in the proximal large bowel.
b. is associated with aortic stenosis.
c. produces a 'corkscrew' appearance of vessels at angiography.
d. is most common at the mesenteric border of bowel.
e. is associated with increased risk of hepatic angiosarcoma.

24. Regarding ischaemic colitis:

a. a mosaic pattern at contrast enema is pathognomonic.
b. affected areas show spasm.
c. stricturing cannot be predicted from the duration of mucosal thumbprinting.
d. affected segments of colon are typically 40–60 cm long.
e. sacculation occurs in areas of stricturing.

25. If, at ultrasound, the liver is less reflective than the adjacent renal parenchyma, the following conditions may be responsible:

a. congestive cardiac failure.
b. cirrhosis.
c. glycogen storage disease type 1.
d. acute hepatitis A.
e. normal variation.

26. **Hepatic iron overload:**

a. causes increased attenuation of the liver parenchyma at unenhanced CT.
b. increases the T2 of liver parenchyma.
c. due to hereditary haemochromatosis is an autosomal recessive trait.
d. increases the reflectivity of the liver at US.
e. increases the risk of hepatic adenoma.

27. **Fibrolamellar carcinoma of the liver:**

a. causes higher serum alpha-fetoprotein levels than hepatocellular carcinoma.
b. is secondary to hepatitis B or C in most cases.
c. frequently shows calcification at CT.
d. has a central scar, which shows delayed enhancement at CT following IV contrast.
e. has a worse prognosis than hepatocellular carcinoma.

28. **Hepatic adenoma:**

a. shows areas of increased attenuation at unenhanced CT.
b. is hypointense at T1-weighted MRI in most cases.
c. is hypervascular at arterial phase CT.
d. shows uptake and excretion into the biliary tree of ^{99m}Tc-HIDA.
e. is characteristically of low reflectivity at US.

29. **Portal vein thrombosis:**

a. complicates acute appendicitis.
b. causes azygos vein enlargement on the chest radiograph.
c. increases the resistive index of the hepatic artery.
d. causes transient hepatic attenuation differences at arterial phase CT.
e. causes the 'spider's web' sign at angiography.

30. **Amoebic abscesses of the liver:**

a. are usually multiple.
b. have thick nodular walls.
c. frequently contain gas at CT.
d. usually occur in the left lobe of liver.
e. often disrupt the diaphragm.

31. Gallbladder carcinoma:

a. is associated with colorectal polyposis.
b. most often appears as gallbladder wall thickening at CT.
c. usually arises from the gallbladder neck.
d. is more common in men.
e. is predisposed to by calcification of the gallbladder wall.

32. Xanthogranulomatous cholecystitis:

a. is predominantly a disease of the elderly.
b. does not extend beyond the gallbladder serosa.
c. is associated with gallstones.
d. produces nodules of increased reflectivity in the gallbladder wall at US.
e. is frequently indistinguishable from gallbladder carcinoma on histology.

33. Adenomyomatosis of the gallbladder:

a. is more common in men.
b. is associated with 'strawberry gallbladder'.
c. results in a 'diamond ring' appearance at US.
d. can be limited to the fundus.
e. is pre-malignant.

34. At MRCP, multifocal strictures of the intrahepatic bile ducts are a feature of:

a. portal vein thrombosis.
b. AIDS cholangiopathy.
c. cholangiocarcinoma.
d. ascending cholangitis.
e. primary biliary cirrhosis.

35. Regarding pancreas divisum:

a. it occurs in 5–10% of the population.
b. the dorsal pancreatic duct drains via the major papilla.
c. CT cannot reliably diagnose this abnormality.
d. there is an association with tracheo-oesophageal fistula.
e. it is a cause of recurrent pancreatitis.

36. Regarding chronic pancreatitis:

a. calcification usually begins at the tail of the pancreas.
b. enlargement of the pancreas is seen at US.
c. pancreatic atrophy is a common finding at CT.
d. intraductal calculi at ERCP indicate marked disease.
e. calcification can lessen as disease progresses.

37. **Regarding cystic neoplasms of the pancreas:**

   a. serous cystadenomas are benign.
   b. serous cystadenomas are hypovascular at arteriography.
   c. the cysts in mucinous cystadenomas are usually larger than 2 cm.
   d. calcification occurs in mucinous cystadenomas.
   e. intraductal papillary mucinous tumours show a predilection for the pancreatic tail.

38. **Splenic infarcts:**

   a. are due to bacterial endocarditis in 70–90%.
   b. occur in polyarteritis nodosa.
   c. are initially of increased reflectivity at US.
   d. show high signal at T1-weighted MRI when haemorrhagic.
   e. are frequently multiple.

39. **Secondary cysts of the spleen:**

   a. are usually post-infective.
   b. are thick-walled at CT.
   c. show rim enhancement at MRI following IV Gd-DTPA.
   d. are commonly septated.
   e. may contain reflective debris at US.

40. **Regarding the spleen:**

   a. a retrorenal spleen occurs in 1.5–2% of people.
   b. accessory spleens are present in 20–30% of the population.
   c. accessory spleens may occur in the thorax.
   d. wandering spleen is more common in women.
   e. splenogonadal fusion only occurs in males.

Module Three: Examination One – Answers

1. Answers

a. **True**
b. **False** – it relaxes the lower oesophageal sphincter, pylorus and duodenum.
c. **False** – small bowel transit time is increased.
d. **True**
e. **True**

(Chapman & Nakielny 2001 p53)

2. Answers

a. **False** – 0.5–5 μm.
b. **True** – to prevent particle clumping.
c. **False** – acidic pH (5.3).
d. **False** – it is an anti-foaming agent.
e. **True** – flocculation is reduced by homogeneous particle size.

(Chapman & Nakielny 2001 pp49–50; Francis et al. p162)

3. Answers

a. **True**
b. **False**
c. **True**
d. **False**
e. **True**

(Chapman & Nakielny 2001 p68)

4. Answers

a. **False** – the phrenicocolic ligament intervenes.
b. **False** – the left space is the larger.
c. **False** – it surrounds the caudate lobe.
d. **True**
e. **True** – the falciform ligament divides the spaces.

(Grainger & Allison pp1142–1144)

5. Answers

a. **True** – the inferior pancreaticoduodenal artery.
b. **False** – D1 = 5 cm, D2 = 7.5 cm, D3 = 10 cm, D4 = 2.5 cm.
c. **False** – anterior to the common bile duct.
d. **True** – in its third part.
e. **False** – posteromedial wall.

(Francis et al. pp56–57)

6. Answers

- **a. True**
- **b. False** – the parotid attenuates between fat and skeletal muscle.
- **c. True**
- **d. False** – sublingual glands are not amenable to sialography.
- **e. True** – demonstrated at parotid sialography.

(Butler et al. pp107–108)

7. Answers

- **a. False** – it is proportional to the square root of the bulk modulus of elasticity.
- **b. False** – it is inversely proportional to the square root of the density.
- **c. True**
- **d. False** – in fat it is 1430 cm s^{-1}, in liver 1580 ms s^{-1}.
- **e. True** – most applications assume a speed of 1540 ms^{-1}.

(Dendy & Heaton pp332–337)

8. Answers

- **a. True**
- **b. False** – increasing frequency increases axial and lateral resolution.
- **c. True**
- **d. True**
- **e. False** – it depends on depth and width of the field of view, the scan-line density and the degree of frame averaging.

(Dendy & Heaton pp346–348)

9. Answers

- **a. True**
- **b. False** – increased signal.
- **c. False** – it is most common in the minor salivary glands of the oral cavity.
- **d. True**
- **e. True**

(Grainger & Allison pp2585–2587; Dähnert pp386 & 390)

10. Answers

- **a. True** – squamous carcinoma develops in patients with longstanding disease, also an achalasia can occur in patients with carcinoma due to destruction of the myenteric plexus.
- **b. False** – an erect swallow.
- **c. False** – hot fluids relieve symptoms.
- **d. False** – they are equally effective.
- **e. True** – hold-up of isotope in the mid-oesophagus is seen on a dynamic study.

(Grainger & Allison pp1024–1025)

11. Answers

- **a. True** – this is the hallmark of a benign submucosal lesion.
- **b. False** – distal third, where the muscularis propria is exclusively smooth muscle.
- **c. False** – only rarely multiple, but has been reported in Alport syndrome.
- **d. True** – it is the only calcifying oesophageal tumour.
- **e. True** – most are asymptomatic due to slow growth.

(Grainger & Allison pp1016–1017)

12. Answers

- **a. True** – although the incidence of adenocarcinoma is increasing, squamous cell tumours still account for 85%.
- **b. True**
- **c. True** – also tobacco smoking.
- **d. True**
- **e. False** – usually of reduced reflectivity.

(Grainger & Allison pp1010–1022)

13. Answers

- **a. True** – they can also occur in the anastomotic ring.
- **b. False** – they are very rare.
- **c. True** – it commonly settles within 2 weeks.
- **d. False** – self-limiting spasm and inflammation are the usual cause.
- **e. True** – in 75% of cases.

(Grainger & Allison p1053; Shaw PC, Op den Orth JO. Post-operative stomach and duodenum. *Radiol Clin North Am* 1994;32:1275–1291)

14. Answers

- **a. False** – there is gastric gland hypertrophy, but achlorhydria.
- **b. False** – the greater curve is the usual site.
- **c. False** – the folds are pliable, distinguishing them from carcinomatous enlargement.
- **d. False** – the antrum is involved in fewer than half of cases.
- **e. True** – due to a protein-losing enteropathy.

(Grainger & Allison pp1046–1047)

15. Answers

- **a. True** – represents preserved gastric mucosa in the ulcer base with undermining of the submucosa.
- **b. True** – this is not seen with malignant ulcers.
- **c. False** – this is a feature of malignancy.
- **d. False** – benign ulcers have smooth, even folds.
- **e. True** – or oval, or round. Malignant ulcers are often irregular.

(Grainger & Allison p1056)

16. Answers

a. **True** – due to increased rate of migration with covered stents.
b. **False** – a nasogastric tube is used to decompress the stomach, improving torque control of the catheters used.
c. **True** – but they are often required to negotiate a tight stricture.
d. **True** – most stents will self-expand over time.
e. **False** – technical success occurs in 94–100%, versus just less than 100% for oesophageal stenting. Clinical success occurs in 80–100%.

(Mauro MA, Koehler RE, Baron TH. Advances in gastrointestinal intervention: the treatment of gastroduodenal and colorectal obstructions with metallic stents. *Radiology* 2000;215:658–669)

17. Answers

a. **False** – relative contraindication.
b. **False** – it can still be performed if a safe subcostal route exists.
c. **False** – towards the fundus.
d. **True** – 5.9% versus 9.4% for endoscopic procedure, 20% for surgery.
e. **True** – it is otherwise an uncommon complication.

(Ho SGF, Marchinkow LO, Legiehn GM et al. Radiological percutaneous gastrostomy. *Clin Radiol* 2001;56:902–910)

18. Answers

a. **True** – they have an enhancing rim and a necrotic core at CT.
b. **False** – lymph node metastases are rare.
c. **True** – metastatic disease is most often to the liver and peritoneum.
d. **True** – ascites is usually seen as a response to treatment.
e. **False** – the tumours expand with a broad, pushing border.

(Burkhill GJC, Backram M, Al-Muderi O et al. Malignant gastrointestinal stromal tumours: Distribution, imaging features, and patterns of metastatic spread. *Radiology* 2003;226:527–532)

19. Answers

a. **False** – the skin rash is urticaria pigmentosa.
b. **True**
c. **False** – they usually occur in short segments of jejunum.
d. **False**
e. **False**

(Grainger & Allison p1094)

20. Answers

a. **True** – nodes have a low attenuation centre in 40–60%.
b. **True**
c. **False** – ascites is typically higher attenuation (20–45 HU).
d. **True**
e. **False** – this occurs in pseudomyxoma peritonei.

(Grainger & Allison pp1456 & 1154)

21. Answers

a. False – epidermoid cysts are a feature of Gardner's syndrome.
b. True – along with skin, breast and thyroid lesions.
c. True – occur following surgery, also in the small bowel mesentery.
d. False – keratoacanthomas are a feature of Torre–Muir syndrome.
e. True – also an increase in ovarian, testicular, breast and pancreatic tumours.

(Grainger & Allison pp1112–1114)

22. Answers

a. True – the sensitivity approaches that of endoscopy.
b. False – phosphosoda produces a drier bowel which improves polyp detection.
c. True – although many findings are of little significance.
d. False – sigmoid distension is better in the prone position.
e. False – stalked polyps can be highly mobile.

(Taylor SA, Halligan S, Bartram CI. CT colonography: Methods, pathology and pitfalls. *Clin Radiol* 2003;58:179–190)

23. Answers

a. True
b. True – in 20%.
c. False – this is a feature of carcinoid syndrome.
d. False – usually the antimesenteric border.
e. False

(Grainger & Allison p1175)

24. Answers

a. False – it also occurs with angioneurotic oedema and herpes zoster.
b. True
c. False – thumbprinting for more than 10 days is associated with increased likelihood of stricture formation.
d. False – usually up to 20 cm.
e. True – on the antimesenteric border; it is also seen in Crohn's disease.

(Grainger & Allison pp1132)

25. Answers

a. True
b. False – cirrhosis increases liver reflectivity.
c. False – this is a cause of increased reflectivity.
d. True – or other causes of acute hepatitis.
e. True

(Dewbury et al. p248)

26. Answers

- **a. True** – the attenuation is typically increased to around 75 HU.
- **b. False** – the T2 is reduced, resulting in signal loss on T2 and T2*-weighted images.
- **c. True**
- **d. True** – though this is non-specific.
- **e. False** – the risk of hepatocellular carcinoma is increased.

(Grainger & Allison pp1249–1250)

27. Answers

- **a. False** – alpha-fetoprotein levels are typically only slightly raised.
- **b. False** – no predisposing causes are known.
- **c. True** – in over half of cases.
- **d. True**
- **e. False** – the prognosis is good, with a 60–70% 5-year survival.

(Grainger & Allison p1263; Dähnert p715)

28. Answers

- **a. True** – due to spontaneous haemorrhage.
- **b. False** – it is often iso- or slightly hyperintense.
- **c. True**
- **d. False** – they take up HIDA, but cannot excrete it as they lack bile ducts.
- **e. False** – it is usually iso- or slightly hyperreflective.

(Grainger & Allison p1258; Dähnert p708)

29. Answers

- **a. True** – also acute pancreatitis, ascending cholangitis.
- **b. True**
- **c. False** – the RI is decreased to less than 0.5 in the acute stage.
- **d. True**
- **e. False** – it causes the 'threads and streaks' sign.

(Dähnert pp736–737)

30. Answers

- **a. False** – solitary.
- **b. True** – 60% of cases.
- **c. False** – not gas containing unless hepatobronchial or hepatoenteric fistula is present.
- **d. False** – right lobe.
- **e. False** – rare, but is strongly suggestive when present.

(Brant & Helms p679; Dähnert p707)

31. Answers

- **a. True**
- **b. False** – a mass replacing the gallbladder is the commonest appearance.
- **c. False** – usually arises at the fundus.
- **d. True**
- **e. True**

(Haaga et al. pp1357–1360)

32. Answers

a. **True** – it is a rare condition seen mainly in the 7th and 8th decades of life.
b. **False** – extension into the pericholecystic fat and liver is seen in almost 50%.
c. **True**
d. **False** – the nodules are of low reflectivity.
e. **False**

(Dähnert p692; Haaga et al. p1353)

33. Answers

a. **False** – three times more common in women.
b. **True** – in one third of cases.
c. **True** – due to comet tail artefacts arising in the thickened gallbladder wall.
d. **True** – producing an umbilicated fundal nodule.
e. **False**

(Grainger & Allison pp1296–1297; Dähnert pp715–716)

34. Answers

a. **False** – hepatic artery thrombosis, following liver transplantation.
b. **True**
c. **True**
d. **True**
e. **True** – also primary sclerosing cholangitis.

(Dähnert pp666–697)

35. Answers

a. **True**
b. **False** – via the minor papilla.
c. **True** – pancreatography is the only way to reliably demonstrate the anomaly.
d. **False** – tracheo-oesophageal fistula is associated with annular pancreas.
e. **True**

(Grainger & Allison p1344; Dähnert p723)

36. Answers

a. **False** – calcification begins in the head of the gland.
b. **True**
c. **True** – 54% in one series.
d. **True**
e. **True** – decalcification is described, but rare.

(Grainger & Allison p1354; Haaga et al. pp1445–1447)

37. Answers

a. **True** – mucinous cystadenomas are pre-malignant.
b. **False** – hypervascular.
c. **True** – in serous cystadenoma, the cysts are more numerous and smaller.
d. **True** – in both mucinous and serous cystadenomas.
e. **False** – more common in the uncinate process of the pancreas.

(Haaga et al. pp1470–1474)

38. Answers

- a. **False** – bacterial endocarditis is the underlying cause in up to 50%.
- b. **True**
- c. **False** – initially of low reflectivity.
- d. **True** – also high signal on T2-weighted MRI with haemorrhage.
- e. **False** – they are more often solitary.

(Dähnert p739; Grainger & Allison p1443; Haaga et al. pp1505–1507)

39. Answers

- a. **False** – usually post-traumatic.
- b. **False** – the wall is thin or imperceptible.
- c. **False** – no enhancement occurs at CT or MRI.
- d. **False** – septation is more common in congenital splenic cysts.
- e. **True**

(Grainger & Allison p1437; Haaga et al. pp1491–1492)

40. Answers

- a. **False** – 15–20%.
- b. **True**
- c. **False** – as opposed to post-traumatic splenosis, which may occur in the thorax.
- d. **True**
- e. **False** – but it is more common in males.

(Grainger & Allison p1436; Haaga et al. pp1488–1489)

Module Three: Examination Two – Questions

1. **Metoclopramide:**

   a. increases lower oesophageal sphincter tone.
   b. relaxes the pyloric antrum.
   c. reduces small bowel transit time.
   d. is contraindicated following recent gastrointestinal haemorrhage.
   e. causes extrapyramidal dystonia more often in elderly patients.

2. **Regarding the contrast swallow:**

   a. a low kV technique is preferred to demonstrate mucosal detail.
   b. aspiration of iopamidol leads to pulmonary oedema.
   c. the water siphon test is used to demonstrate gastro-oesophageal reflux.
   d. acquisition at 4–6 frames s^{-1} is adequate for assessment of the hypopharynx.
   e. varices are best demonstrated in the prone RPO position.

3. **In the investigation of diseases of the salivary glands:**

   a. suppurative sialadenitis is an indication for sialography.
   b. Lipiodol Ultrafluid causes less pain at sialography than water-soluble iodinated contrast.
   c. sialoscintigraphy is performed using ^{99m}Tc-DTPA.
   d. sialography is indicated in the investigation of a parotid mass.
   e. magnetic resonance sialography uses heavily T2-weighted sequences.

4. **With respect to the radiological anatomy of the stomach:**

   a. the 'magenstrasse' is a mucosal fold paralleling the lesser curve.
   b. gastric rugae are normally 3–5 mm thick.
   c. areae gastricae are most prominent in the gastric body.
   d. the incisura angularis occurs on the lesser curve.
   e. the transverse mesocolon is a posterior relation at CT.

5. **Regarding the anatomy of the colon:**

   a. the ascending colon is usually intraperitoneal.
   b. the descending colon is wider than the ascending colon.
   c. haustra are more prominent in the ascending than descending colon.
   d. the transverse colon is related anteriorly to the greater omentum.
   e. the splenic flexure is usually more caudal than the hepatic flexure.

6. **The common bile duct:**

   a. can indent the first part of the duodenum at barium meal.
   b. is dilated if its diameter is 7 mm in a 30-year-old woman at US.
   c. is closely related to the superior mesenteric artery.
   d. usually lies anterior to the hepatic artery at the porta hepatis.
   e. lies anterior to the foramen of Winslow.

7. **Helical CT:**

   a. can only be performed on fourth generation scanners.
   b. has a pitch inversely proportional to collimated slice thickness.
   c. has reduced motion artefact relative to conventional axial CT.
   d. allows for reduced dose by increasing pitch.
   e. permits reconstruction at slice thicknesses less than the beam collimation at the detectors.

8. **The following are true of MRI:**

   a. the gyromagnetic ratio of protons depends on the field strength of the magnet.
   b. T2* dephasing occurs more slowly than T2 dephasing.
   c. The T1 of a tissue is longer than its T2.
   d. the longitudinal component of magnetisation is responsible for the received signal.
   e. the net magnetisation vector precesses at the Larmor frequency in the static magnetic field, B_0.

9. **Concerning oesophageal motility:**

   a. primary peristalsis is a stripping wave that traverses the entire oesophagus.
   b. primary peristalsis is initiated by distension of the oesophageal lumen.
   c. tertiary peristalsis starts in the mid-oesophagus and spreads up and down.
   d. tertiary peristalsis causes the appearance of a 'corkscrew oesophagus'.
   e. secondary peristalsis are non-productive contractions.

10. **Epiphrenic diverticula of the oesophagus:**

   a. occur just above the lower oesophageal sphincter.
   b. usually occur on the left side.
   c. are a common incidental finding at barium swallow.
   d. are usually found in patients with oesophageal motility disorders.
   e. have a large, wide-mouthed neck.

11. Concerning malignant lesions of the oesophagus:

a. leiomyosarcomas are aggressive lesions, which metastasise early.
b. primary oesophageal melanoma has a poor prognosis.
c. breast carcinoma is the commonest source of metastases to the distal oesophagus.
d. primary oesophageal carcinoma accounts for 25–30% of GI malignancies.
e. dysphagia is the commonest presenting symptom.

12. Oesophageal webs:

a. are usually located just distal to the cricopharyngeal impression.
b. are thin membranes that sweep partially across the lumen.
c. are frequently multiple.
d. typically arise from the posterior wall.
e. cause dysphagia.

13. Regarding duodenal ulcers:

a. they are associated with acid hypersecretion.
b. most occur on the superior wall of the duodenal bulb.
c. post-bulbar ulcers represent approximately 5% of the total.
d. ulcer craters have no mucosal lining.
e. perforations tend to occur more frequently along the posterior wall.

14. Adenomatous gastric polyps:

a. over 2 cm are malignant in most cases.
b. are more common than gastric carcinoma.
c. are frequently multiple.
d. do not occur in familial adenomatous polyposis.
e. most often occur in the antrum.

15. Gastric involvement in Crohn's disease:

a. occurs in 10–20%.
b. usually occurs in the absence of ileal disease.
c. is usually associated with duodenal involvement.
d. causes a 'cobblestone' appearance of the mucosal pattern.
e. spares the antrum in most cases.

16. Regarding gastric leiomyomas:

a. ulceration of the overlying mucosa is a rare feature.
b. most lesions show calcification at CT.
c. they appear as submucosal nodules on barium studies.
d. a 'bull's eye' appearance is due to ulceration.
e. most lesions are extramural.

17. Coeliac disease:

a. is associated with squamous carcinoma of the oesophagus.
b. causes villous atrophy, most marked in the distal small bowel.
c. can be reliably diagnosed by enteroclysis.
d. causes small bowel dilatation.
e. is associated with non-obstructive intussusception.

18. Concerning metastases to the small bowel:

a. haematogenous spread occurs along the mesenteric border.
b. haematogenous spread is the commonest route of dissemination.
c. intraperitoneal implantation of the serosa is commonly due to ovarian carcinoma in women.
d. malignant melanoma spreads haematogenously.
e. barium studies demonstrate nodules, and tethering of folds.

19. Small bowel carcinoid tumour:

a. most frequently occurs in the ileum.
b. produces a desmoplastic reaction in the mesentery.
c. characteristically shows early filling of veins at angiography.
d. causes stricturing.
e. causes the carcinoid syndrome in 20–30%.

20. Lymphoma of the small bowel:

a. can be the presenting feature of coeliac disease.
b. is more common in the jejunum than the ileum.
c. causes cavitating ulcers.
d. does not cause shouldered strictures.
e. produces aneurysmal dilatation of the small bowel.

21. Hereditary nonpolyposis colorectal carcinoma:

a. usually affects the rectosigmoid colon.
b. has an increased incidence of synchronous colorectal cancers.
c. is prevalent in 1% of patients with colorectal carcinomas.
d. is more common than familial adenomatous polyposis.
e. of the Lynch I subtype is associated with extracolonic malignancies.

22. Regarding the diagnosis of colorectal tumours at barium enema:

a. carpet lesions are most common in the transverse and descending colon.
b. most carcinomas appear as annular or semi-annular lesions.
c. polypoid lesions rarely occur in the caecum.
d. rectal lesions are frequently annular.
e. synchronous colorectal carcinomas are present in 20–30%.

23. **Concerning ulcerative colitis:**

a. the ileocaecal valve is often thickened.
b. colonic strictures are a recognised complication.
c. lead-pipe colon is a feature of chronic disease.
d. widening of the presacral space occurs.
e. colonic adenocarcinoma is the commonest cause of death.

24. **Features of diverticular disease include:**

a. shortening of the bowel.
b. localisation of diverticula in the proximal colon in fewer than 1%.
c. frequent involvement of the rectum.
d. diverticulitis is more common in the transverse colon than the caecum.
e. enlargement of diverticula at barium enema during episodes of colitis.

25. **Focal fatty change of the liver:**

a. assumes a geometric pattern.
b. often shows some enhancement at CT following IV contrast.
c. extends to the periphery of the liver.
d. may cause displacement of vessels and mass effect.
e. is commonly found adjacent to the falciform ligament.

26. **MRI features of hepatocellular carcinoma include:**

a. a high signal capsule on T1-weighted images.
b. heterogeneously increased signal on T2-weighted images.
c. a relative reduction in signal intensity following IV ferrumoxide.
d. a central low attenuation scar on T2-weighted images.
e. early enhancement following IV Gd-DTPA.

27. **With respect to focal nodular hyperplasia:**

a. most tumours have a central fibrous scar.
b. high velocity Doppler signals with arterial pulsatility may be seen.
c. it is clearly perceptible as a focal lesion on non-contrast CT.
d. the central scar is of high signal on T2-weighted MRI.
e. the margin of the mass is usually well-defined.

28. **Regarding hydatid disease of the liver:**

a. calcification of the outer cyst wall implies death of the parasite.
b. the cyst septa enhance on CT following IV contrast.
c. the risk of anaphylaxis following percutaneous aspiration is 30–50%.
d. the 'water lily' sign on US is characteristic.
e. the septa are of high signal on T1-weighted MRI.

29. **48 hours after orthotopic liver transplantation, the following imaging findings are considered normal:**

a. periportal oedema at CT.
b. a left pleural effusion.
c. a fluid collection in the lesser sac at CT.
d. a parvus tardus waveform of the hepatic artery.
e. subhepatic haematoma.

30. **At MRI, the following liver lesions can exhibit a central scar:**

a. hepatocellular carcinoma.
b. fibrolamellar carcinoma.
c. adenoma.
d. focal nodular hyperplasia.
e. haemangioma.

31. **Concerning extrahepatic cholangiocarcinomas:**

a. they comprise 10–30% of all cases of cholangiocarcinoma.
b. Klatskin tumours occur near the junction of the right and left bile ducts.
c. most cases present with an intraductal polypoid mass.
d. the majority are anaplastic carcinomas.
e. biliary cirrhosis is a recognised complication.

32. **Regarding acalculous cholecystitis:**

a. there is an association with polyarteritis nodosa.
b. gallbladder wall thickening is less marked than in calculous cholecystitis.
c. Murphy's sign is typically absent.
d. infection with *Salmonella typhi* is a recognised cause.
e. ^{99m}Tc-HIDA scintigraphy is normal in most cases.

33. Regarding congenital abnormalities of the gallbladder:

a. the gallbladder is absent in 0.025%.
b. absence of the gallbladder is associated with Hirschsprung's disease.
c. a double gallbladder is of no clinical significance.
d. a Phrygian cap deformity is associated with chronic cholecystitis.
e. 10% of gallbladders have a long mesentery.

34. Regarding sclerosing cholangitis:

a. it is associated with ulcerative colitis in 45–55% of cases.
b. portal triads are poorly seen on US.
c. biliary cirrhosis is a recognised complication.
d. duct diverticula demonstrated at cholangiography are pathognomonic.
e. the cystic duct is almost always involved.

35. In the imaging of acute pancreatitis:

a. US shows reduced reflectivity of the gland.
b. CT to stage severity is best performed 48–72 hours after onset.
c. slight variation in pancreatic enhancement from head to tail at CT is normal.
d. gas bubbles within an area of necrosis are pathognomonic of infection.
e. CT appearances correlate well with morbidity and mortality.

36. CT signs of unresectability of pancreatic carcinoma include:

a. extension of the tumour beyond the margins of the pancreas.
b. tumour involvement of adjacent organs.
c. enlarged regional nodes to larger than 15 mm.
d. encasement or obstruction of peripancreatic arteries or veins.
e. ascites.

37. Regarding the pancreatic manifestations of von Hippel–Lindau disease:

a. cysts occur in most cases.
b. microcystic adenomas occur in fewer than 10%.
c. gadolinium enhancement of septations distinguishes microcystic adenoma from a cluster of simple cysts at MRI.
d. islet cell tumours are of low signal at T2-weighted MRI.
e. phaeochromocytoma occurs more frequently in patients with islet cell tumours.

38. **Polysplenia:**

   a. is characterised by multiple small spleens in the left abdomen.
   b. is usually fatal before one year of age.
   c. is associated with situs ambiguus.
   d. is associated with bilateral trilobed lungs.
   e. is associated with left isomerism.

39. **Splenic angiosarcoma:**

   a. rarely metastasises.
   b. is associated with previous exposure to Thorotrast.
   c. is associated with exposure to vinyl chloride.
   d. appears as low attenuation nodules containing haemorrhage at CT.
   e. has a generally indolent course.

40. **Concerning the spleen in lymphoma:**

   a. primary splenic lymphoma is rare.
   b. splenomegaly in lymphoma is benign in one third of cases.
   c. lesions can calcify before treatment.
   d. focal lesions are more common in Hodgkin's than non-Hodgkin's lymphoma.
   e. lymphomatous lesions enhance poorly at CT following IV contrast.

Module Three: Examination Two – Answers

1. Answers

a. **True**
b. **True** – also the duodenal cap.
c. **True** – increases small bowel peristalsis.
d. **True**
e. **False** – more common in young women.

(Francis et al. p165)

2. Answers

a. **False** – barium work requires high kV.
b. **False** – iopamidol (Gastromiro) is non-ionic water soluble contrast.
c. **True**
d. **True**
e. **True**

(Grainger & Allison p1006, p1012; Chapman & Nakielny 2001 p56)

3. Answers

a. **False** – it is a contraindication.
b. **True** – but it is no longer used due to risk of foreign body granulomas following extravasation.
c. **False** – ^{99m}Tc-pertechnetate is used.
d. **False** – there is no indication for evaluation of the ducts with parotid tumours.
e. **True**

(Chapman & Nakielny 2001 pp333–335; Grainger & Allison pp2582–2583)

4. Answers

a. **True** – most pronounced on the erect views of a barium meal.
b. **True**
c. **False** – most prominent in the antrum.
d. **True**
e. **True**

(Francis et al. p54)

5. Answers

a. **False** – the ascending colon only has a mesentery in 10–15% of people.
b. **False** – the ascending colon is wider.
c. **True**
d. **True**
e. **False** – the splenic flexure is usually more cranial.

(Butler et al. pp217–218)

6. Answers

- a. **True**
- b. **True** – 5 mm is the upper limit of normal for young patients.
- c. **False**
- d. **True**
- e. **True**

(Butler et al. pp251–252; Dähnert p676)

7. Answers

- a. **False** – both third and fourth generation scanners can be used.
- b. **True**
- c. **True** – due to faster scan times.
- d. **True**
- e. **False** – this is not possible.

(Dendy & Heaton pp267–270; Farr & Allisy-Roberts p114; Haaga et al. pp8–9)

8. Answers

- a. **False** – it is a property of the nucleus.
- b. **False** – it occurs more rapidly, due to field inhomogeneities.
- c. **True**
- d. **False** – it is the transverse magnetisation that produces the signal.
- e. **False** – individual protons precess but the net vector does not, due to lack of phase coherence between protons.

(Hashemi & Bradley pp32–48)

9. Answers

- a. **True**
- b. **False** – secondary peristalsis.
- c. **False** – secondary peristalsis.
- d. **True**
- e. **False** – tertiary peristalsis.

(Brant & Helms p709)

10. Answers

- a. **True**
- b. **False** – right side.
- c. **False** – rare.
- d. **True**
- e. **False** – narrow neck, which may trap food and liquids and cause symptoms.

(Brant & Helms p712)

11. Answers

- a. **False**
- b. **True**
- c. **True**
- d. **False** – only 7%.
- e. **True**

(Grainger & Allison pp1016–1023)

12. Answers

a. **True** – but may occur anywhere.
b. **True**
c. **False** – only occasionally multiple.
d. **False** – anterior wall.
e. **True**

(Brant & Helms p716; Dähnert p820)

13. Answers

a. **True**
b. **False** – anterior wall in 50%, superior wall only 5%.
c. **True** – majority involve the second and third parts of the duodenum, which are frequently narrowed.
d. **True** – therefore no mucosal relief pattern; do not contract with peristalsis.
e. **False** – anterior wall.

(Brant & Helms p733; Dähnert p814)

14. Answers

a. **True**
b. **False**
c. **False** – usually solitary lesions.
d. **False** – seen in association with hyperplastic polyps in this condition.
e. **True**

(Grainger & Allison pp1054–1055)

15. Answers

a. **True**
b. **False** – ileocolic disease is commonly present.
c. **True** – duodenal involvement alone is more common than gastric disease.
d. **True**
e. **False** – the antrum and body are almost always involved.

(Grainger & Allison pp1045–1046)

16. Answers

a. **False** – occurs in approximately 50% of cases.
b. **False** – 4% of lesions are calcified.
c. **True**
d. **True** – responsible for significant bleeding.
e. **False** – intraluminal submucosal in 60%.

(Brant & Helms p727; Dähnert p840)

17. Answers

- **a. True** – also increased risk of small bowel lymphoma, adenocarcinoma and pharyngeal carcinoma.
- **b. False** – it is most marked in the jejunum.
- **c. False** – the radiological findings are non-specific.
- **d. True** – also 'jejunisation' of the ileum, and total effacement of the jejunal mucosal pattern.
- **e. True** – producing a 'coiled spring' appearance.

(Grainger & Allison p1082)

18. Answers

- **a. False** – antimesenteric border, where submucosal vessels arborise.
- **b. False** – peritoneal seeding is most common.
- **c. True** – colon, pancreatic and gastric carcinoma in men.
- **d. True**
- **e. True** – due to mesenteric fibrosis.

(Brant & Helms pp740–741)

19. Answers

- **a. True** – 90% of small bowel carcinoid occurs here.
- **b. True**
- **c. False** – the veins do not fill, a stellate arterial pattern is seen.
- **d. True**
- **e. False** – it only occurs in 2% of patients with tumours.

(Grainger & Allison p1084; Haaga et al. pp1196–1197)

20. Answers

- **a. True** – rarely, coeliac disease is usually diagnosed some 10 years earlier.
- **b. False** – except in lymphoma associated with alpha chain disease.
- **c. True**
- **d. False** – shouldering is an occasional feature.
- **e. True** – a characteristic finding, which occurs in the absence of a stricture.

(Grainger & Allison p1085)

21. Answers

- **a. False** – 70% are proximal to the splenic flexure.
- **b. True**
- **c. False** – 10% of patients.
- **d. True** – 5 times more common.
- **e. False** – Lynch II is associated with extracolonic malignancies, e.g. TCC of ureters; Lynch I is not associated with extracolonic malignancies.

(Dähnert pp805–806)

22. Answers

a. **False** – carpet lesions are most common in the rectum, caecum and ascending colon.
b. **True** – 53% annular/semi-annular, 38% polypoid and 9% plaque-like.
c. **False** – polypoid lesions are most common in the rectum and caecum.
d. **False** – due to the calibre of the rectum, annular lesions are rare.
e. **False** – synchronous carcinomas in 5%, polyps in over one third. Metachronous carcinomas occur in 5%.

(Levine MS, Rubesin SE, Laufer I et al. Diagnosis of colorectal neoplasms at double-contrast barium enema examination. *Radiology* 2000;216:11–18)

23. Answers

a. **False** – not usually thickened but gaping.
b. **True** – 10% of cases.
c. **True** – rigid symmetrical narrowing of colon.
d. **True** – in the acute stage.
e. **False** – toxic megacolon.

(Brant & Helms pp757–758; Dähnert pp863–864)

24. Answers

a. **True** – due to elastin deposition in the taenia coli.
b. **False** – this occurs in 10%.
c. **False** – rectal diverticular disease is rare.
d. **False** – most common in the sigmoid, rare in the caecum, very rare in the transverse colon.
e. **False** – loss of muscle tone closes the neck of diverticula, so they 'disappear' on barium enemas.

(Grainger & Allison pp1119–1123)

25. Answers

a. **True**
b. **False** – no contrast enhancement.
c. **True**
d. **False** – does not cause a mass effect.
e. **True**

(Brant & Helms pp670–671; Dähnert pp702–703)

26. Answers

a. **False** – the capsule is of low signal.
b. **True**
c. **False** – HCC does not take up ferrumoxide, and so becomes more prominent against a low signal background of normal liver.
d. **True**
e. **True** – paralleling the hypervascular CT enhancement pattern.

(Grainger & Allison p1262)

27. Answers

a. **True** – on CT, MRI and US.
b. **True** – due to arteriovenous shunts.
c. **False** – barely perceptible.
d. **True**
e. **False** – usually ill-defined but occasionally shows a capsule.

(Brant & Helms pp677–678; Dähnert pp703–704)

28. Answers

a. **False** – all cyst layers must be calcified to infer the death of the parasite.
b. **True** – the cyst wall also enhances.
c. **False** – anaphylactic shock occurs in 0.5%.
d. **True** – but rare.
e. **False** – the septa are low signal on T1- and T2-weighted sequences.

(Grainger & Allison p1253; Dähnert p700)

29. Answers

a. **True**
b. **False** – right pleural effusions are a normal finding.
c. **True**
d. **True** – usually due to oedema at the hepatic artery anastomosis. In most cases the parvus tardus waveform resolves.
e. **True**

(Dähnert p717)

30. Answers

a. **True**
b. **True**
c. **True**
d. **True**
e. **True**

(Grainger & Allison p1256; Dähnert p715)

31. Answers

a. **False** – 90%.
b. **True**
c. **False** – 5% of cases – causes stenosis or obstruction of the CBD in most cases.
d. **False** – 11% are anaplastic, the majority are adenocarcinoma.
e. **True** – secondary to obstruction.

(Brant & Helms pp682–683; Dähnert pp704–705)

32. Answers

a. **True**
b. **False**
c. **False**
d. **True** – very rare, actinomycosis is even rarer.
e. **False**

(Grainger & Allison p1295; Dähnert p691)

33. Answers

- **a. True**
- **b. False** – associations with imperforate anus, rectovaginal fistula and absent scapula and radius.
- **c. False** – the second gallbladder is frequently diseased.
- **d. True** – due to biliary stasis and cholelithiasis.
- **e. True** – predisposes them to torsion and herniation into the lesser sac.

(Grainger & Allison pp1277–1278; Haaga et al. pp1345–1346; Dähnert pp677–678)

34. Answers

- **a. True**
- **b. False** – brightly reflective.
- **c. True**
- **d. True** – pseudodiverticula occur.
- **e. False** – involved in approximately 15% of cases.

(Brant & Helms pp681–682)

35. Answers

- **a. True** – also generalised or focal enlargement of the gland.
- **b. True**
- **c. True** – but it is usually less than 30 HU difference.
- **d. False** – gas may also arise from fistulation to the GI tract.
- **e. True** – using Balthazar's CT Severity Index.

(Grainger & Allison pp1348–1351; Balthazar EJ. Acute pancreatitis: Assessment of severity with clinical and CT evaluation. *Radiology* 2002;223:603–613)

36. Answers

- **a. True**
- **b. True**
- **c. True**
- **d. True**
- **e. True**

(Brant & Helms pp693–695)

37. Answers

- **a. False** – they occur in 40%.
- **b. True** – 4%.
- **c. True**
- **d. False** – they are of high signal, and appear as low signal on fat-suppressed T1 sequences.
- **e. True**

(Tattersall DJ, Moore NR. Von Hippel-Lindau disease: MRI of abdominal manifestations. *Clin Radiol* 2002;57:85–92)

38. Answers

a. False – usually located in the right abdomen.
b. False – a feature of asplenia.
c. True
d. False – this occurs with asplenia.
e. True

(Brant & Helms p700)

39. Answers

a. False – liver metastases occur in 70%.
b. True – also to arsenic.
c. True
d. True
e. False – it is an aggressive lesion with a poor prognosis.

(Grainger & Allison p1440; Haaga et al. p1491)

40. Answers

a. True – 1–2% of all lymphoma.
b. True
c. True – rarely.
d. False – more common in non-Hodgkin's.
e. True

(Grainger & Allison p1440; Haaga et al. pp1489–1490)

Module Three: Examination Three – Questions

1. **Glucagon:**

   a. is given as a 1 mg dose for a barium meal.
   b. has a slower onset of action than hyoscine N-butylbromide.
   c. is a more potent smooth muscle relaxant than hyoscine N-butylbromide.
   d. is contraindicated in patients with type 2 diabetes.
   e. increases small bowel transit time.

2. **Concerning the double-contrast barium examination of the stomach and duodenum:**

   a. gastrointestinal haemorrhage is a contraindication.
   b. 300–500 ml of gas is sufficient.
   c. no patient preparation is required.
   d. hyoscine N-butylbromide reduces the sensitivity for hiatus hernia.
   e. demonstration of the areae gastricae indicates adequate mucosal coating.

3. **The radionuclide detection of Meckel's diverticulum:**

   a. utilises ^{99m}Tc-tin colloid.
   b. should not be undertaken within 3 days of a small bowel meal.
   c. does not require any patient preparation.
   d. uses intravenous ranitidine to inhibit the secretion of tracer by gastric mucosa.
   e. requires the field of view to be restricted to the lower abdomen and pelvis.

4. **The gastroduodenal artery:**

   a. arises from the common hepatic artery in most people.
   b. passes anterior to the first part of the duodenum.
   c. gives rise to the posterior superior pancreaticoduodenal artery.
   d. gives rise to the anterior superior pancreaticoduodenal artery.
   e. gives blood supply to the common bile duct.

5. **Regarding the anatomy of the oesophagus:**

   a. it is 40 cm long.
   b. it traverses the diaphragm at the level of T10.
   c. the right vagus nerve lies anteriorly.
   d. it is attached to the diaphragm by Laimer's fascia.
   e. the A ring represents the gastro-oesophageal junction.

6. **Concerning the adult pancreas:**

   a. it lies in the anterior pararenal space.
   b. the gland slopes caudally from head to tail.
   c. the tail lies in the gastrosplenic ligament.
   d. it is of greater reflectivity than the liver at US.
   e. the uncinate lobe is of different reflectivity to the head of the pancreas at US.

7. **Regarding US transducers:**

   a. the bandwidth increases as pulse length decreases.
   b. the efficiency of US production is optimal above the Curie temperature.
   c. the thickness of the piezoelectric transducer is equal to twice the wavelength of the transmitted beam.
   d. the lens lies between the piezoelectric transducer and the matching layer.
   e. the backing layer is incorporated to reduce 'ringing'.

8. **The presence of the following are contraindications to MRI:**

   a. dynamic hip screw.
   b. Bjork–Shiley prosthetic heart valve.
   c. cochlear implant.
   d. cholecystectomy clips inserted 4 weeks ago.
   e. embolisation coils in the inferior mesenteric artery inserted 8 weeks ago.

9. **Salivary calculi:**

   a. are most common in the sublingual glands.
   b. are a common feature of Sjögren's syndrome.
   c. are radio-opaque in 20–40%.
   d. may cause sialectasis at sialography.
   e. cause strictures of the submandibular duct.

10. **Regarding systemic sclerosis:**

   a. absent peristalsis is seen in the proximal third of the oesophagus.
   b. it is characterised by hypertrophy of the smooth muscle of the bowel wall.
   c. the oesophagus collapses on emptying.
   d. intussusception of the small bowel is a recognised complication.
   e. the oesophagus is affected in most patients.

11. Transverse oesophageal mucosal folds are seen at barium swallow in:

a. achalasia.
b. scleroderma.
c. reflux oesophagitis.
d. corrosive oesophagitis.
e. feline oesophagus.

12. Regarding oesophageal perforation:

a. upper oesophageal perforations usually cause a left-sided hydrothorax.
b. most cases are due to spontaneous rupture following forceful vomiting.
c. distal perforations due to forceful vomiting usually occur at the right posterior lateral wall.
d. soft tissue emphysema develops within 1 hour of perforation.
e. mortality varies between 3% and 5%.

13. The following CT findings favour a diagnosis of gastric carcinoma rather than gastric lymphoma:

a. obliteration of the perigastric fat planes.
b. regional lymphadenopathy.
c. lymphadenopathy below the level of the renal veins.
d. duodenal involvement.
e. wall thickening less than 4 cm.

14. Gastric volvulus:

a. is most often of the mesenteroaxial type.
b. is associated with phrenic nerve palsy.
c. is predisposed to by gastric distension.
d. is only rarely associated with hiatus hernia.
e. characteristically presents with projectile vomiting.

15. Gastric varices:

a. are usually seen with oesophageal varices.
b. seen in isolation are a sign of splenic vein thrombosis.
c. require maximal distension of the stomach at double-contrast barium meal if they are to be detected.
d. often occur in the antrum alone.
e. may mimic the appearance of gastric lymphoma.

16. **Concerning benign conditions of the duodenum:**

a. Crohn's disease affects the duodenum in 20–30%.
b. involvement in systemic sclerosis is unusual.
c. intramural haematomas are more common in the elderly.
d. traumatic rupture typically occurs at the junction of the first and second parts.
e. Bouveret's syndrome has a high mortality rate.

17. **Concerning the CT manifestations of Crohn's disease:**

a. mesenteric lymphadenopathy is a feature.
b. fibrofatty proliferation of the mesentery is the commonest finding.
c. abscesses contain gas in most cases.
d. if disease is limited to the mucosa, CT is often normal.
e. mural stratification of thickened bowel wall indicates acute disease.

18. **Regarding small bowel neoplasms:**

a. primary carcinoma is more common in the jejunum than the ileum.
b. chronic myeloid leukaemia predisposes to small bowel lymphoma.
c. leiomyomas produce a tumour blush at angiography.
d. leiomyosarcomas enhance poorly on CT following IV contrast.
e. carcinoid causes thickening of the valvulae conniventes.

19. **Involvement of the small bowel by systemic sclerosis causes:**

a. increased mucosal folds at barium follow through.
b. decreased gut transit time.
c. pseudodiverticula.
d. jejunal strictures.
e. duodenal dilatation.

20. **Regarding infection and infestation of the small bowel:**

a. giardiasis thickens the valvulae conniventes in the duodenum.
b. absence of jejunal valvulae occurs in strongyloidiasis.
c. abdominal actinomycosis occurs most often in the jejunum.
d. tuberculosis causes 'cobblestoning' of the terminal ileum.
e. small bowel obstruction occurs in ascariasis.

21. Regarding acute colitides:

a. total colonic involvement is a feature of pseudomembranous colitis.
b. ischaemic colitis rarely affects the splenic flexure.
c. abdominal radiographs are normal in most cases of pseudomembranous colitis.
d. free perforation occurs rarely in Crohn's disease.
e. the transverse colon may normally measure up to 75 mm.

22. Solitary rectal ulcer syndrome:

a. is due to prolapse of the posterior rectal wall.
b. is associated with a large intake of spicy foods.
c. causes strictures.
d. evacuation proctography demonstrates failure of anorectal angle to open on straining.
e. is a pre-malignant condition.

23. Regarding CT and the diagnosis of acute appendicitis:

a. CT has resulted in a decrease in negative appendicectomies.
b. oral contrast reduces the sensitivity for appendicoliths.
c. extraluminal air is a specific feature for perforation.
d. an extraluminal appendicolith has a high sensitivity for perforation.
e. a defect in the enhancing appendiceal wall is a non-specific finding.

24. With respect to endometriosis and the colon:

a. implants are most common on the caecum.
b. defects are frequently multiple and of variable size.
c. barium studies demonstrate filling defects that usually encircle the colon.
d. CT demonstrates a complex cystic pelvic mass with high density fluid components.
e. implants are of low signal at T1-weighted MRI.

25. The following US findings are suggestive of portal hypertension:

a. portal vein diameter of 10 mm.
b. reverse flow in the right portal vein, and normal flow in the left branch.
c. portal vein velocity of 6 cm s^{-1} at Doppler US.
d. recanalisation of the umbilical vein.
e. increase in portal venous flow during inspiration.

26. If, on unenhanced CT, the liver is of increased attenuation, the cause may be:

a. Wilson's disease.
b. glycogen storage disease.
c. previous exposure to Thorotrast.
d. treatment with triiodo-thyronine.
e. amyloidosis.

27. Metastases to the liver:

a. from caecal tumours are more common in the right lobe.
b. usually take their blood supply from the portal vein.
c. in the absence of a known primary, are most often from lung carcinoma.
d. from the thyroid are hypervascular.
e. are multiple in most cases.

28. Haemangiomas of the liver:

a. are associated with hereditary haemorrhagic telangiectasia.
b. enlarge during pregnancy.
c. show centrifugal progression of enhancement at MRI.
d. are usually of increased reflectivity on US.
e. should not be biopsied, due to the risk of haemorrhage.

29. Regarding Budd–Chiari syndrome:

a. damping of the hepatic vein Doppler waveform is non-specific.
b. the liver is of reduced attenuation at unenhanced CT.
c. sulphur colloid scintigraphy shows photopaenia of the caudate lobe.
d. hepatic vein thrombus is of high signal at T1-weighted spin-echo MRI.
e. a 'thread and streaks' appearance at venography is characteristic.

30. Pyogenic liver abscesses:

a. commonly present with jaundice.
b. are distinguished from a simple cyst by their lack of posterior enhancement at US.
c. show peripheral enhancement at CT following IV contrast.
d. are photopaenic at ^{99m}Tc-sulphur colloid scintigraphy.
e. are of high signal at T2-weighted MRI.

31. **Cholangiocarcinoma:**

a. is more often extrahepatic than intrahepatic.
b. is of reduced attenuation at unenhanced CT.
c. is of increased signal at T1-weighted MRI.
d. does not enhance following IV Gd-DTPA.
e. is often of reduced reflectivity at US.

32. **AIDS causes the following abnormalities of the biliary tract:**

a. diffuse thickening of the gallbladder wall and bile ducts.
b. cholangitis due to *Mycobacterium avium intracellulare.*
c. stricturing of the distal common bile duct.
d. ulceration of the common bile duct.
e. cholesterolosis of the gallbladder.

33. **Regarding porcelain gallbladder:**

a. oral cholecystography shows a non-functioning gallbladder.
b. Rokitansky–Aschoff sinuses are a feature.
c. it is associated with gallstones in 80–90% of cases.
d. it carries a 10–20% risk of gallbladder carcinoma.
e. cholecystectomy is indicated.

34. **Concerning stent insertion for biliary strictures due to cholangiocarcinoma:**

a. metallic stents are preferable if there is marked tumour invasion of the duodenum.
b. metallic stents cannot be removed.
c. balloon-expandable stents are preferable to self-expanding stents.
d. covered stents offer no significant increase in patency rates to non-covered stents.
e. the 12-month patency rate is greater for hilar than non-hilar obstruction.

35. **Pancreatic pseudocysts:**

a. are most common in the lesser sac.
b. usually form within 10 days of onset of pancreatitis.
c. can undergo spontaneous haemorrhage.
d. are better drained by a transgastric than an external route.
e. are best drained between 6 and 12 weeks.

36. **The following statements concerning islet cell tumours are true:**

a. lesions containing calcifications are usually benign.
b. diarrhoea is a feature of gastrinomas.
c. non-functioning islet cell tumours are usually 4 mm to 4 cm at presentation.
d. gastrinomas are of high signal at fat-suppressed T2-weighted MRI.
e. 80–90% of non-functioning tumours are malignant.

37. **Regarding the CT features of pancreatic ductal carcinoma:**

a. an obstructed CBD typically shows gradual narrowing.
b. most tumours are poorly enhancing following IV contrast.
c. tumour calcification is present in most cases.
d. dilatation of the posterior superior pancreaticoduodenal vein indicates venous invasion by tumour.
e. ascites occurs in fewer than 20%.

38. **Peliosis:**

a. occurs in HIV infection.
b. is more common in the liver than the spleen.
c. cannot be demonstrated at US.
d. causes multiple low attenuation lesions in the spleen at CT.
e. may reverse on withdrawal of the causative drugs.

39. **Splenic abscesses:**

a. are due to anaerobic bacteria in most instances.
b. contain gas at CT in 20–30%.
c. show peripheral enhancement at CT following IV contrast.
d. are of low reflectivity at US.
e. are secondary to endocarditis in the majority.

40. **Splenic hamartomas:**

a. are usually solitary.
b. rarely cause symptoms.
c. are of low signal at T2-weighted MRI.
d. are of increased reflectivity at US.
e. are photopaenic at ^{99m}Tc-sulphur colloid scintigraphy.

Module Three: Examination Three – Answers

1. Answers

a. **False** – 0.1–0.3 mg is sufficient for barium meal, 1 mg is the dose for colonic relaxation in barium enema.
b. **True** – approximately 1 minute.
c. **True**
d. **False**
e. **False** – no effect.

(Chapman & Nakielny 2001 p54)

2. Answers

a. **False** – it is an indication, although it may confound later radionuclide studies and angiography.
b. **True**
c. **False** – the patient should be fasted for 6 hours and desist from smoking cigarettes.
d. **False**
e. **True**

(Chapman & Nakielny 2001 pp57–58; Grainger & Allison pp1036–1037)

3. Answers

a. **False** – ^{99m}Tc-pertechnetate.
b. **True** – residual barium attenuates 140 keV gamma photons from ^{99m}Tc.
c. **False** – a 6-hour fast is needed.
d. **True**
e. **False** – the stomach must be included in the images.

(Chapman & Nakielny 2001 pp99–100)

4. Answers

a. **True** – in 75%, it may also arise from the left hepatic, right hepatic or superior mesenteric arteries.
b. **False** – it passes posteriorly.
c. **True**
d. **True**
e. **True**

(Butler et al. pp229–230)

5. Answers

a. **False** – 25 cm long – the gastro-oesophageal junction is 40 cm from the incisor teeth.
b. **True**
c. **False** – the left vagus is anterior, the right posterior.
d. **True** – also called the phreno-oesophageal ligament.
e. **False** – it is the proximal extent of the phrenic ampulla.

(Grainger & Allison pp1005–1006)

6. Answers

- **a. True**
- **b. False** – the tail is cranial to the head.
- **c. False** – the tail lies in the lienorenal ligament.
- **d. True**
- **e. True** – it is often of lower reflectivity than the head.

(Butler et al. pp253–255)

7. Answers

- **a. True** – bandwidth in MHz is the reciprocal of pulse length in μs.
- **b. False** – the piezoelectric crystal loses its properties above the Curie temperature.
- **c. False** – half the wavelength.
- **d. False** – the lens is placed beyond the matching layer.
- **e. True**

(Dendy & Heaton pp339–341)

8. Answers

- **a. False**
- **b. False**
- **c. True**
- **d. False**
- **e. False**

(Westbrook & Kaut pp239–241)

9. Answers

- **a. False** – calculi are most common in the submandibular glands.
- **b. False**
- **c. False** – most salivary calculi are radio-opaque.
- **d. True**
- **e. True**

(Grainger & Allison p2583)

10. Answers

- **a. False** – distal two-thirds.
- **b. False** – smooth muscle undergoes atrophy and fibrosis.
- **c. False** – tends to remain dilated.
- **d. True**
- **e. True**

(Brant & Helms pp710–711; Dähnert pp853–855)

11. Answers

- **a. True** – but this is uncommon.
- **b. True**
- **c. True**
- **d. True** – uncommon.
- **e. True**

(Reeder p619)

12. Answers

a. **False** – right sided.
b. **False** – majority due to instrumentation.
c. **False** – left posterior lateral wall.
d. **True**
e. **False** – 20% and 60%.

(Brant & Helms pp719–721)

13. Answers

a. **True** – the fat planes are usually preserved in lymphoma.
b. **False** – this is common in both.
c. **False** – lymphadenopathy does not extend below this level in carcinoma.
d. **False** – this is seen in both, but is not common.
e. **True** – lymphoma often produces diffuse, marked thickening of the gastric wall. In carcinoma the mean wall thickness is 1.8 cm.

(Grainger & Allison p1058)

14. Answers

a. **False** – organo-axial volvulus is more common.
b. **True**
c. **True**
d. **False** – it usually occurs in the presence of a hiatus hernia.
e. **False** – there is classically violent retching, but little or no vomitus.

(Grainger & Allison pp1047–1048)

15. Answers

a. **True**
b. **True**
c. **False** – over-distension reduces the sensitivity for varices.
d. **False** – only rarely.
e. **True**

(Grainger & Allison p1051)

16. Answers

a. **False** – 4%.
b. **False** – it is commonly involved.
c. **False** – usually seen in children.
d. **False** – most often at the junction of the second and third parts.
e. **True** – this is gastric outlet obstruction by gallstones.

(Grainger & Allison pp1070–1073)

17. Answers

a. **True** – they are usually 3–8 mm in short axis diameter.
b. **False** – bowel wall thickening is the commonest finding.
c. **False** – only in 30–50% (abscesses occur in 15–20%).
d. **True**
e. **True**

(Grainger & Allison pp1081–1082; Haaga et al. pp1203–1204)

18. Answers

- **a. True** – it is only rarely found in the ileum.
- **b. False** – chronic lymphatic leukaemia is a risk factor, however.
- **c. True**
- **d. False** – they have a strongly enhancing rim.
- **e. True**

(Grainger & Allison pp1083–1085)

19. Answers

- **a. True** – 'hidebound' appearance.
- **b. False** – transit time is increased due to reduced peristalsis.
- **c. True** – square sacculations with a broad base.
- **d. False** – jejunal dilatation occurs.
- **e. True**

(Grainger & Allison p1093)

20. Answers

- **a. True** – causes irregular thickening of the valvulae.
- **b. True** – the valvulae conniventes may also be thickened.
- **c. False** – the appendix is the commonest abdominal site.
- **d. False** – this helps distinguish it from Crohn's disease.
- **e. True** – if a sufficient number of worms are present.

(Grainger & Allison pp1087–1088)

21. Answers

- **a. True**
- **b. False**
- **c. True** – abnormalities are present in one third.
- **d. True**
- **e. False** – dilatation greater than 55 mm is significant.

(Grainger & Allison pp988–990)

22. Answers

- **a. False** – anterior rectal wall, causing mucosal ischaemia.
- **b. False**
- **c. True**
- **d. True**
- **e. False**

(Dähnert p859)

23. Answers

- **a. True**
- **b. True**
- **c. True** – but it has a poor sensitivity.
- **d. False** – the sensitivity of this finding is only 20.5%.
- **e. False** – it is 100% specific for perforation, with a sensitivity of 64%.

(Horrow MH, White DS, Horrow JC. Differentiation of perforated from non-perforated appendix at CT. *Radiology* 2003;227:46–57)

24. Answers

a. **False** – sigmoid colon and rectum.
b. **True**
c. **False** – indents but does not usually encircle the colon.
d. **True**
e. **False** – high signal at T1-weighting.

(Brant & Helms p756)

25. Answers

a. **False** – 13 mm or greater. SMV or splenic vein diameter of greater than 10 mm is suggestive.
b. **True** – this occurs with 'steal' of right portal flow by recanalised umbilical vein.
c. **True** – normal portal vein velocity is 12–30 cm s^{-1}.
d. **True** – paraumbilical veins recanalise in 20–35% of cases.
e. **False** – this is a normal phenomenon, which is lost in portal hypertension.

(Brant & Helms p673; Dähnert pp733–734)

26. Answers

a. **True**
b. **True**
c. **True**
d. **False** – amiodarone treatment does increase liver attenuation, however.
e. **False** – amyloidosis can reduce liver attenuation.

(Reeder p692)

27. Answers

a. **True** – due to streaming via the right portal vein branch – left colonic lesions show no lobar predilection, however.
b. **False** – metastases are supplied by the hepatic artery in most cases.
c. **False** – the colon is the source in 42%, the lung in 14%.
d. **True**
e. **True** – multiple in 50–98%.

(Grainger & Allison p1254; Dähnert p720)

28. Answers

a. **True**
b. **True** – sometimes.
c. **False** – enhancement progresses centripetally, and can take up to 30 minutes to fill in with large lesions.
d. **True** – unless they are large, when reflectivity may be reduced.
e. **False** – biopsy is safe providing normal liver intervenes between the lesion and the liver capsule.

(Grainger & Allison p1254; Dähnert p710)

29. Answers

a. **True** – also seen in cirrhosis.
b. **True** – due to congestive oedema.
c. **False** – the caudate appears as an area of relatively increased activity.
d. **True** – if it is less than 5 weeks old.
e. **False** – a 'spider's web' appearance is characteristic; 'threads and streaks' describes the appearance of portal vein thrombosis.

(Grainger & Allison pp1266–1267; Dähnert pp683–684)

30. Answers

a. **False** – jaundice occurs in up to 20%.
b. **False** – abscesses also show posterior acoustic enhancement.
c. **True** – peripheral enhancement may not occur following antibiotic therapy.
d. **True** – they appear as 'hot spots' on ^{67}Ga- or ^{111}In-leucocyte studies.
e. **True**

(Grainger & Allison pp1253–1254; Dähnert pp707–708)

31. Answers

a. **True**
b. **True**
c. **False** – low signal.
d. **False**
e. **False** – usually of increased reflectivity.

(Dähnert pp685–687; Haaga et al. pp1378–1383)

32. Answers

a. **True**
b. **True** – more often due to *Cryptosporidium* and cytomegalovirus.
c. **True**
d. **True**
e. **False**

(Dähnert p688; Haaga et al. pp1365–1366)

33. Answers

a. **True**
b. **True**
c. **True**
d. **True**
e. **True** – due to risk of developing carcinoma (occurs in 10–20%).

(Brant & Helms pp686 & 840; Dähnert p732)

34. Answers

- **a. False** – this is an indication for a plastic stent.
- **b. True**
- **c. False** – self-expanding stents are less rigid, and so easier to deploy around a curve.
- **d. True**
- **e. False** – following metallic stent insertion, the 12-month patency for hilar obstruction is 46%, and for non-hilar obstruction 89%.

(Hatzidakis A, Adam A. The interventional radiological management of cholangiocarcinoma. *Clin Radiol* 2003;58:91–96)

35. Answers

- **a. False** – most common in and immediately around the pancreas.
- **b. False** – pseudocysts take several weeks to mature.
- **c. True**
- **d. True**
- **e. True** – before 6 weeks some pseudocysts will resolve spontaneously, after 13 weeks the rate of infection, rupture and bleeding increase.

(Haaga et al. pp1437–1445 & 2205–2208)

36. Answers

- **a. False** – calcifications are highly suggestive of malignancy.
- **b. True** – due to gastric hypersecretion.
- **c. False** – tend to be much larger (6–20 cm).
- **d. True**
- **e. True**

(Brant & Helms pp695–697; Dähnert pp724–726)

37. Answers

- **a. False** – the CBD usually comes to an abrupt halt as it is occluded by tumour.
- **b. True**
- **c. False** – calcification is rare, seen in approximately 2%.
- **d. True**
- **e. True** – ascites is seen in 7–10%.

(Dähnert p724; Haaga et al. pp1458–1462)

38. Answers

- **a. True** – due to infection with *Bartonella henselae*.
- **b. True**
- **c. False** – ill-defined areas of mixed reflectivity occur.
- **d. True**
- **e. True** – peliosis may also be caused by anabolic steroids.

(Dähnert p732; Haaga et al. pp1498–1499)

39. Answers

a. **False** – *E. coli*, *Staphylococcus* and *Salmonella* cause most cases.
b. **False** – splenic abscesses only rarely contain gas.
c. **True** – enhancement may be absent.
d. **True** – or anechoic.
e. **True**

(Grainger & Allison p1441; Haaga et al. pp1495–1496)

40. Answers

a. **True** – they are rare lesions of the spleen.
b. **True** – may cause pain, anorexia, pancytopaenia and weight loss.
c. **False** – hyperintense at T2- and hypointense at T1-weighted MRI.
d. **True** – may have cystic areas.
e. **False** – hamartomas show uptake of sulphur colloid tracer.

(Grainger & Allison p1440; Haaga et al. pp1494–1495)

MODULE FOUR

Genitourinary, Obstetrics and Gynaecology, and Breast

Time Allowed: 2 hours

Module Four: Examination One – Questions

1. **Concerning the geometry of the transmitted US beam:**

   a. the length of the near field increases with increasing frequency.
   b. the length of the near field is independent of the size of the transducer.
   c. the degree of divergence in the far field is increased by reducing transducer frequency.
   d. the beam can be focussed with an electromagnetic lens.
   e. increasing the curvature of the piezoelectric transducer reduces the focal length.

2. **In MRI, increasing TR has the following effects:**

   a. decreased acquisition time.
   b. reduced T1-weighting.
   c. increased signal-to-noise ratio.
   d. increased proton density weighting.
   e. reduction in the number of slices that can be acquired.

3. **Regarding congenital renal anomalies:**

   a. ectopic kidneys are more common on the left.
   b. renal agenesis is more common on the right.
   c. unilateral renal agenesis has an incidence of 1 in 1000.
   d. horseshoe kidneys have an incidence of 1 in 2000.
   e. with malrotation, upper pole calyces are medial to lower pole calyces.

4. **Regarding the IVU:**

   a. the nephrographic density is independent of the glomerular filtration rate.
   b. myeloma is a contraindication to low osmolar contrast.
   c. prone positioning can improve ureteric filling.
   d. the compression band must be removed to perform oblique views.
   e. the optimal swing angle for tomography is 8–10 degrees.

5. **In the imaging of a patient with primary hyperaldosteronism:**

   a. most cases are due to adrenal hyperplasia.
   b. MRI is the modality of choice.
   c. adenomas are usually less than 2 cm.
   d. with adrenal hyperplasia, CT is normal in one third.
   e. IV contrast is mandatory for CT.

6. **Adrenal metastases:**

a. are most commonly from breast cancer.
b. occur in half of cases of malignant melanoma.
c. characteristically occur to the adrenal medulla.
d. show persistent contrast enhancement at delayed CT.
e. appear heterogeneous at CT.

7. **Concerning adrenal 'incidentalomas':**

a. they are found in 5–10% of abdominal CT examinations.
b. most adrenal lesions larger than 6 cm are malignant.
c. in patients with lung cancer, half of all adrenal lesions are benign.
d. MRI can distinguish functioning from non-functioning adenomas.
e. attenuation less than 35 HU at delayed contrast-enhanced CT is diagnostic of an adenoma.

8. **Regarding diseases of the penis:**

a. carcinomas are most often of the squamous cell type.
b. carcinoma metastasises late to local lymph nodes.
c. carcinoma spreads early via the haematogenous route.
d. the inguinal nodes are spared in advanced disease.
e. Peyronie's disease is seen as highly reflective plaques at US.

9. **Concerning scrotal scintigraphy:**

a. the patient is positioned standing.
b. ^{99m}Tc-DTPA is utilised.
c. a slow injection of radioisotope is needed.
d. activity is increased in epididymo-orchitis.
e. a photon-deficient area is seen in ischaemia.

10. **Regarding carcinoma of the prostate:**

a. it usually begins in the peripheral zone.
b. the histology is transitional cell carcinoma in 10–20%.
c. it is commonly isoreflective at transrectal US.
d. transrectal US is sensitive for seminal vesicle invasion.
e. extracapsular extension often occurs via the neurovascular bundles.

11. Chronic prostatitis:

a. is usually due to *E. coli*.
b. causes elongation of the prostatic urethra at MCUG.
c. is associated with urethral strictures.
d. due to tuberculosis results in cavitation at MCUG.
e. can be distinguished from prostate cancer at transrectal US.

12. A pear-shaped bladder at IVU is a recognised feature of:

a. lymphoma.
b. trauma.
c. spina bifida.
d. pelvic lipomatosis.
e. amyloidosis.

13. Regarding the use of MRI in bladder carcinoma imaging:

a. lesions smaller than 1 cm cannot be reliably detected.
b. tumour is of lower signal than normal bladder wall on T1-weighted images.
c. TNM T1 disease can be differentiated from T2 disease.
d. bone metastases are most conspicuous on T2-weighted sequences.
e. MRI is superior to CT in staging advanced disease.

14. With mechanical bladder disorders:

a. trabeculation is seen in bladder outlet obstruction.
b. trabeculation is not seen in a neurogenic bladder.
c. diverticula are more common in females.
d. bladder herniae have a wide neck.
e. descent of any part of the bladder to the level of the superior pubic ramus during straining indicates a cystocoele.

15. Urethral strictures:

a. are often neoplastic in origin.
b. follow gonococcal urethritis.
c. of inflammatory origin are most common in the post-bulbar urethra.
d. commonly occur in tuberculosis.
e. are associated with seronegative arthropathy.

16. **In the ultrasound diagnosis of renal calculi:**

a. the lowest available frequency should be used.
b. the gain should be turned down low.
c. stone composition is an important factor.
d. stone size is underestimated.
e. examination in varying positions does not improve sensitivity.

17. **Regarding angiomyolipomas:**

a. 70–80% arise in patients with tuberous sclerosis.
b. they are associated with neurofibromatosis.
c. no fat attenuation is present at CT in 5%.
d. acoustic shadowing occurs at US.
e. a high signal capsule at T2-weighted MRI is a recognised feature.

18. **Xanthogranulomatous pyelonephritis:**

a. usually involves the kidney diffusely.
b. is associated with a renal calculus in the majority.
c. does not extend beyond the kidney.
d. shows rim enhancement at CT following IV contrast.
e. is best treated by nephrostomy.

19. **Renal oncocytomas:**

a. frequently appear necrotic at CT.
b. appear photopaenic at ^{99m}Tc-DMSA scintigraphy.
c. appear as homogenous masses on US.
d. commonly show calcification at CT.
e. are best diagnosed by needle biopsy.

20. **The following findings at CT indicate unresectability of renal cell carcinoma:**

a. fat stranding and increased collateral vessels in the perinephric space.
b. a maximum tumour diameter of 11 cm.
c. an enhancing filling defect in the IVC.
d. liver metastases.
e. para-aortic lymph nodes with a 2 cm short axis diameter.

21. **Pyeloureteritis cystica:**

a. is most common in the bladder.
b. is usually unilateral.
c. causes haematuria.
d. increases the risk of transitional cell carcinoma.
e. is a cause of infundibular stenosis at IVU.

22. Concerning the investigation of urinary calculi with unenhanced helical CT:

a. stones of all compositions are readily demonstrated.
b. CT is poor at demonstrating the central lucency of phleboliths.
c. prone scanning is of no proven benefit.
d. fat stranding is more common around the kidney than the ureter.
e. increased attenuation of the medullary pyramids indicates obstruction.

23. Regarding MRI of the female pelvis:

a. the endometrium is of high signal on T2-weighted images.
b. the endometrium enhances following IV Gd-DTPA.
c. IUCDs are a contraindication.
d. the parametrium is of low signal on T1-weighted images.
e. contraceptive diaphragms produce artefact.

24. Concerning hysterosalpingography:

a. it is best performed in the second half of the menstrual cycle.
b. iso-osmolar water soluble contrast media is used.
c. venous intravasation has a significant morbidity.
d. pethidine is suitable analgesia for any discomfort during the examination.
e. the uterus should be visualised en face.

25. Oligohydramnios is associated with the following conditions:

a. prune belly syndrome.
b. omphalocoele.
c. post-maturity.
d. premature rupture of membranes.
e. rhesus incompatibility.

26. Gastroschisis:

a. is associated with normal cord insertion.
b. commonly involves the liver.
c. is associated with fetal ascites.
d. causes intra-uterine growth restriction.
e. has a poorer prognosis than omphalocoele.

27. Antenatal US features of neural tube defects include:

a. a lemon-shaped cerebellum.
b. microcephaly.
c. flattening of the skull at the level of the coronal sutures.
d. increased nuchal thickness.
e. spinal irregularity with an overlying skin defect.

28. **The following are major US criteria of pregnancy failure:**

a. a 6 mm embryo without a heartbeat at transabdominal US.
b. a gestation sac of 20 mm without an embryo.
c. the absence of growth after 7–10 days.
d. an irregular contour of the gestation sac.
e. the empty amnion sign.

29. **Regarding mature cystic teratoma of the ovary:**

a. a fat–fluid level at CT is diagnostic.
b. tumours can be entirely cystic, with no solid elements.
c. the average size is 20 cm at presentation.
d. elevation of serum alpha-fetoprotein occurs.
e. malignant degeneration is not a feature.

30. **US features suggestive of ovarian malignancy include:**

a. solid areas of high reflectivity in a mass.
b. thick nodular septations.
c. size greater than 7 cm.
d. peripheral vascularity.
e. a resistive index less than 0.6.

31. **Regarding the appearance of the endometrium:**

a. the thickness should not be more than 4 mm post menopause.
b. polyps are multiple in most cases.
c. hyperplasia is a precursor to carcinoma.
d. transvaginal US is the modality of choice for assessment of endometrial carcinoma.
e. polyps typically measure from 5 to 15 mm.

32. **Hydatidiform mole:**

a. is associated with hypothyroidism.
b. is excluded by finding a live fetus at transvaginal US.
c. appears as a highly reflective uterine mass as transvaginal US.
d. is associated with theca lutein cysts.
e. degenerates into choriocarcinoma.

33. **Regarding plain film findings with gynaecological pathology:**

a. a fat–fluid level is pathognomonic of a dermoid cyst.
b. popcorn calcification suggests pseudomyxoma peritonei.
c. uterine tube calcification is suggestive of tuberculosis.
d. bone destruction by gynaecological tumours is rarely seen.
e. plain films are the investigation of choice to check IUCD position.

34. Concerning endometriosis:

a. 'shading' may be seen at T1-weighted MRI.
b. fat suppression improves the detection of endometriomas with MRI.
c. bladder wall involvement is common.
d. high signal is seen in multiple cysts at T1-weighted MRI.
e. cyst septation is uncommon.

35. Regarding mammography:

a. a 0.3 mm molybdenum filter is used.
b. a small focal spot is required.
c. a film-focus distance of 1 meter is standard.
d. double-sided film is used.
e. a kVp of 26–30 kV is used.

36. Regarding lymph node involvement in breast cancer:

a. 40% of women have axillary lymphadenopathy at diagnosis.
b. involved nodes are rounder and more reflective than normal at US.
c. internal mammary nodes are more often involved than the axillary nodes in tumours of the inner quadrants of the breast.
d. internal mammary nodes are usually resected at mastectomy.
e. supraclavicular nodal spread confers a poor prognosis.

37. The following can appear as a stellate lesion at mammography:

a. fat necrosis.
b. fibroadenoma.
c. galactocoele.
d. radial scar.
e. breast cyst.

38. Concerning male breast cancer:

a. most cases occur in patients with Klinefelter's syndrome.
b. it is frequently bilateral.
c. mammographic calcifications are fewer than in female breast cancer.
d. it is more common on the left.
e. gynaecomastia is a predisposing factor.

39. **Breast biopsy:**

a. US-guided biopsy is preferred to stereotactic biopsy for masses.
b. US-guided biopsy is preferred to stereotactic biopsy for microcalcifications.
c. the patient lies prone for stereotactic biopsy.
d. needles of 14 gauge or larger should be used for wide-bore core biopsy.
e. vacuum-assisted biopsy yields greater amounts of tissue.

40. **Regarding benign breast disease:**

a. breast abscesses are most commonly located in the upper-outer quadrant.
b. breast abscesses are most commonly due to *Streptococcus*.
c. skin retraction is a common presentation of fat necrosis.
d. traumatic fat necrosis forms a spiculated density.
e. hyalinised fibroadenomas are common.

Module Four: Examination One – Answers

1. Answers

a. **True**
b. **False** – it is proportional to the square of the radius of the piezoelectric transducer.
c. **True** – higher frequency probes have narrower far fields.
d. **False**
e. **True**

(Dendy & Heaton pp341–343)

2. Answers

a. **False** – increased in proportion with TR.
b. **True**
c. **True**
d. **True**
e. **False** – increases the number that can be acquired per TR.

(Hashemi & Bradley p171)

3. Answers

a. **True**
b. **False** – more common on the left.
c. **True**
d. **False** – 1 in 400.
e. **False** – this is the normal orientation, with malrotation the upper pole calyces lie more laterally.

(Dewbury et al. pp525–527; Grainger & Allison pp1720–1721)

4. Answers

a. **False** – it depends on GFR, plasma concentration of contrast, and tubular reabsorption of water and sodium.
b. **False** – it is an indication; high osmolar contrast is contraindicated.
c. **True**
d. **False**
e. **False** – 8–10 degrees for zonography, 25–30 degrees for tomography.

(Chapman & Nakielny 2001 pp142–143)

5. Answers

a. **False** – 70% are due to adrenocortical adenomas.
b. **False** – CT is preferred for its better spatial resolution.
c. **True**
d. **True**
e. **False** – the aim of imaging is to distinguish between hyperplasia and adenoma, for which contrast is unnecessary.

(Haaga et al. pp1514–1517)

6. Answers

a. **False** – lung is the commonest source.
b. **True**
c. **False** – they occur to the corticomedullary junction.
d. **True**
e. **True** – a necrotic centre with a rim of enhancement.

(Haaga et al. pp1526–1528; Dähnert p928)

7. Answers

a. **False** – 0.5–1.5%.
b. **True**
c. **True** – but 30–40% are metastases.
d. **False** – this is the role of biochemistry.
e. **True**

(Haaga et al. p1525; Dähnert p910)

8. Answers

a. **True**
b. **False** – early nodal metastasis.
c. **False** – late.
d. **False** – drainage is to these nodes.
e. **True**

(Sutton pp1033–1034)

9. Answers

a. **False** – supine.
b. **True**
c. **False** – rapid bolus injection.
d. **False** – normal.
e. **True**

(Sutton pp1034–1035)

10. Answers

a. **True** – in 70%.
b. **False** – 95% are adenocarcinomas.
c. **False** – it is of low reflectivity in 60%, and isoreflective in 35%.
d. **False** – 100% specificity but only 29% sensitivity.
e. **True**

(Grainger & Allison pp1637–1641; Dähnert pp939–941; Haaga et al. pp1724–1726)

11. Answers

a. **True** – or *Staphylococcus*.
b. **True** – the urethra is also narrowed and straightened.
c. **True**
d. **True** – in advanced cases.
e. **False** – TRUS is painful, and adds little to the diagnosis.

(Grainger & Allison pp1633–1634)

12. Answers

a. **True** – due to pelvic lymphadenopathy.
b. **True** – due to pelvic haematoma.
c. **False**
d. **True**
e. **False**

(Dähnert p887)

13. Answers

a. **True**
b. **False** – same signal as normal bladder wall.
c. **True**
d. **False** – T1-weighted sequences.
e. **False** – MRI is similar to CT in advanced disease; it is superior in early disease.

(Sutton pp1009–1011)

14. Answers

a. **True**
b. **False** – trabeculation is a feature of neurogenic bladder.
c. **False** – males.
d. **False** – narrow neck.
e. **False** – the level of the pubic ramus.

(Sutton pp993–994)

15. Answers

a. **False** – most are inflammatory or post-traumatic.
b. **True**
c. **True**
d. **False** – only 2% of cases.
e. **True** – strictures occur in Reiter's disease.

(Sutton pp1017–1018)

16. Answers

a. **False** – the highest frequency should be used.
b. **True** – to increase shadowing.
c. **False** – diagnosis is independent of composition on US.
d. **False** – stone size is overestimated.
e. **False** – this improves sensitivity.

(Dewbury et al. pp579–580)

17. Answers

a. **False** – 80% are sporadic, 20% occur in tuberous sclerosis.
b. **True** – also von Hippel–Lindau syndrome.
c. **True**
d. **True** – in one third.
e. **False** – the lesions do not have capsules.

(Grainger & Allison pp1565–1566; Dähnert pp912–913; Haaga et al. pp1577–1578)

18. Answers

a. **True** – in 85–90%; the focal form is less common.
b. **True** – 70%.
c. **False** – it can extend to the perinephric fat, psoas, colon and skin.
d. **True** – it may mimic renal cell carcinoma, particularly if focal.
e. **False** – nephrectomy is the usual treatment.

(Grainger & Allison pp1551–1552; Dähnert pp944–945; Haaga et al. pp1585–1586)

19. Answers

a. **False** – necrosis is not often seen at CT.
b. **True** – they do not take up DMSA.
c. **True**
d. **False** – rare.
e. **False** – biopsy may miss the disease; frozen section at time of surgery is employed.

(Dewbury et al. pp557–558; Dähnert pp933–934)

20. Answers

a. **False** – these findings occur in stage II (and sometimes stage I) disease.
b. **False** – tumour size is not a determining factor.
c. **False** – stage IIIA disease may still undergo surgery.
d. **True** – stage IV disease is inoperable.
e. **False** – stage IIIB disease.

(Haaga et al. p1561)

21. Answers

a. **True** – also occurs in proximal ureter and pelviureteric junction.
b. **True**
c. **True** – it is frequently asymptomatic.
d. **True**
e. **False** – multiple 1–3 mm filling defects in the collecting system occur at IVU.

(Grainger & Allison pp1553–1554; Dähnert p945)

22. Answers

a. **False** – all stones except those due to HIV protease inhibitors, e.g. indinavir.
b. **True**
c. **False** – it can help differentiate bladder calculi from VUJ calculi.
d. **True** – periureteral stranding is rarely seen without perinephric stranding.
e. **False** – the absence of dense pyramids is a secondary sign of obstruction.

(Dähnert p982; Haaga et al. pp1599–1601; Sutton pp965–971)

23. Answers

a. **True**
b. **True**
c. **False** – safe
d. **False** – intermediate signal.
e. **True**

(Sutton p1093)

24. Answers

- **a. False** – first half.
- **b. True**
- **c. False** – no clinical significance.
- **d. False** – it causes tubal spasm.
- **e. True**

(Sutton pp1085–1086)

25. Answers

- **a. True**
- **b. False** – polyhydramnios
- **c. True**
- **d. True**
- **e. False** – associated with polyhydramnios.

(Dähnert pp989–990)

26. Answers

- **a. True**
- **b. False** – the liver does not often herniate out.
- **c. False** – it is associated with polyhydramnios.
- **d. True**
- **e. False** – better prognosis.

(Dähnert p1037)

27. Answers

- **a. False** – banana-shaped cerebellum, lemon-shaped skull.
- **b. True** – also dolichocephaly.
- **c. True**
- **d. False**
- **e. True**

(Dewbury et al. vol. 3 pp284–285)

28. Answers

- **a. False** – 6 mm at transvaginal US, 10 mm at transabdominal scanning.
- **b. False** – a 20 mm sac without a yolk sac, or 25 mm without an embryo.
- **c. True**
- **d. False** – this sign is unreliable, present in only 10%.
- **e. True** – this is identification of an amnion without an embryonic pole.

(Dewbury et al. vol. 3 pp170–171)

29. Answers

- **a. True**
- **b. True**
- **c. False** – the average size at diagnosis is 10 cm.
- **d. False**
- **e. False** – it occurs in 1–3%.

(Dähnert pp1027–1028; Haaga et al. p1734)

30. Answers

a. **False** – low reflectivity is a feature.
b. **True**
c. **True**
d. **False** – central vascularity.
e. **True** – a RI of > 0.8 suggests benignity.

(Sutton p1083)

31. Answers

a. **True**
b. **False** – multiple in 20%.
c. **True**
d. **False** – MRI is.
e. **True**

(Sutton pp1077–1078; Dähnert p1004)

32. Answers

a. **False** – hyperthyroidism may occur due to beta-hCG, however.
b. **False** – a fetus may coexist with hydatidiform mole in 1–2%.
c. **True** – containing cystic spaces in many cases.
d. **True**
e. **True**

(Grainger & Allison p2213; Dähnert p1039)

33. Answers

a. **True**
b. **False** – it is a feature of fibroids.
c. **True**
d. **True**
e. **False** – US is the preferred method.

(Sutton p1085)

34. Answers

a. **False** – shading is a phenomenon seen on T2-weighted images.
b. **True**
c. **False** – it is uncommon.
d. **True** – due to blood products.
e. **False**

(Dähnert pp1032–1034; Sutton pp1079–1080; Haaga et al. pp1779–1781; Brant & Helms p824)

35. Answers

a. **False** – 0.03 mm molybdenum filter.
b. **True**
c. **False** – 60–65 cm film-focus distance.
d. **False** – single-sided.
e. **True**

(Sutton p1451)

36. Answers

a. **True**
b. **False** – larger, rounder and less reflective than normal lymph nodes.
c. **False** – axillary nodes are still the commonest site of spread.
d. **False**
e. **True**

(Husband & Reznek pp404–405)

37. Answers

a. **True**
b. **True**
c. **False**
d. **True**
e. **False**

(Reeder p840)

38. Answers

a. **False** – 4% occur in patients with Klinefelter's syndrome.
b. **False**
c. **True** – and rounder, larger and more scattered.
d. **True**
e. **False**

(Dähnert pp556–557)

39. Answers

a. **True** – where they can be confidently seen on US.
b. **False**
c. **True**
d. **True**
e. **True** – and so should produce greater diagnostic accuracy.

(The Royal College of Radiologists. *Guidance on screening and symptomatic breast imaging.* 2nd edn. 2003; Grainger and Allison pp2264–2265)

40. Answers

a. **False** – most often retroareolar.
b. **False** – staphylococcal in most cases.
c. **True**
d. **True**
e. **False** – they are rare.

(Grainger and Allison p2252)

Module Four: Examination Two – Questions

1. **Concerning contrast agents used in US:**

   a. they consist of microbubbles of nitrogen.
   b. 0.1–1% of the intravenous dose lodges in the pulmonary capillary bed.
   c. augmentation of the US signal persists for up to 15–20 minutes.
   d. they remain confined to the blood pool following injection.
   e. they are contraindicated in acute renal failure.

2. **Regarding the male urethra:**

   a. it is narrowest in the prostatic segment.
   b. the ejaculatory ducts open onto the verumontanum.
   c. the glands of Cowper open onto the membranous urethra.
   d. blood supply is via branches of the obturator artery.
   e. the penile urethra is surrounded by the corpus spongiosum.

3. **Concerning the testes:**

   a. the epididymis lies on the posteromedial surface.
   b. lymphatic drainage occurs to the external iliac nodes.
   c. the vas deferens crosses posterior to the external iliac artery.
   d. the right testicular vein drains into the right renal vein.
   e. the mediastinum testis runs transversely.

4. **The following are true of dynamic renal scintigraphy:**

   a. ^{99m}Tc-DTPA is excreted by tubular secretion.
   b. ^{99m}Tc-MAG 3 allows the measurement of glomerular filtration rate.
   c. ^{99m}Tc-glucoheptonate can be used for dynamic imaging.
   d. normal drainage is confirmed if renal activity reduces by more than 50% after IV furosemide.
   e. the radiation dose is lower than for an IVU.

5. **Concerning adrenal calcification:**

   a. tuberculosis is the commonest cause.
   b. it is a feature of Wolman's disease.
   c. it occurs in ganglioneuromas.
   d. pseudocysts are the commonest calcified masses in adults.
   e. histoplasmosis is a recognised cause.

6. **Adrenal myelolipomas:**
   a. are at risk of malignant degeneration.
   b. do not calcify.
   c. reach sizes of 30 cm.
   d. arise from smooth muscle elements in the adrenal.
   e. are characteristically of homogenous attenuation at CT.

7. **Regarding phaeochromocytoma:**
   a. it is usually less than 5 cm at diagnosis.
   b. the pancreas is the commonest site for extra-adrenal tumours.
   c. calcification is seen at CT.
   d. marked enhancement occurs following IV contrast.
   e. it is of high signal at T1-weighted MRI.

8. **Regarding benign scrotal disease:**
   a. scrotal cysts are most common in adolescence.
   b. epididymal cysts are more common at the upper pole.
   c. epidermoid cysts appear hyperaemic at colour Doppler.
   d. varicocoeles are commoner on the right.
   e. the post-vasectomy vas is usually atrophic.

9. **The following are true of testicular tumours:**
   a. they are of high signal at T2-weighted MRI.
   b. MRI features reliably differentiate benign from malignant lesions.
   c. metastasis is commonly to the internal iliac and inguinal lymph nodes.
   d. haematogenous spread occurs early with choriocarcinoma.
   e. tumours disrupt the normal parenchymal septations.

10. **In benign prostatic hypertrophy:**
    a. the central zone of the prostate hypertrophies.
    b. there is detrusor hypertrophy.
    c. symptoms are closely related to bladder volume.
    d. transrectal US shows cystic change.
    e. prostatic calcification occurs.

11. **Regarding MRI of prostate cancer:**
    a. tumour is usually of low signal at T2-weighting.
    b. signal intensity of the prostate correlates with the amount of glandular spaces.
    c. post-biopsy change can persist for several months.
    d. seminal vesicle invasion is best assessed at T1-weighting.
    e. staging accuracy is significantly improved by an endorectal coil.

12. **Schistosomiasis of the urinary tract:**

   a. is typically caused by *Schistosoma mansoni.*
   b. results in hyperperistaltic ureters.
   c. causes beaded stenosis of the ureters.
   d. produces poor bladder emptying secondary to calcification in the wall.
   e. results in a rapid onset of renal disease.

13. **Acquired bladder diverticula:**

   a. are more common than congenital diverticula.
   b. occur in Ehlers–Danlos syndrome.
   c. are more common in women.
   d. are associated with increased risk of bladder carcinoma.
   e. are multiple in 5–20%.

14. **Regarding the bladder:**

   a. cystitis cystica occurs largely in diabetics.
   b. intraluminal gas is a feature of bacterial cystitis.
   c. bladder calculi are usually composed of struvite or urate.
   d. fungal cystitis causes filling defects at IVU.
   e. filling defects due to malakoplakia are most common at the bladder dome.

15. **Concerning abnormalities at ascending urethrography:**

   a. post-traumatic strictures are usually short.
   b. luminal irregularity is a feature of Reiter's syndrome.
   c. amyloidosis causes intraluminal filling defects.
   d. schistosomiasis is associated with reflux into Cowper's glands.
   e. inflammatory strictures are most common in the penile urethra.

16. **Regarding renal vein thrombosis:**

   a. dehydration is a common cause in adults.
   b. it occurs in 20–35% of patients with the nephrotic syndrome.
   c. it causes a striated nephrogram at IVU.
   d. corticomedullary differentiation is lost at CT following IV contrast.
   e. thrombus is of high signal at T1-weighted gradient echo MRI.

17. Concerning tuberculosis of the urinary tract:

a. most patients do not have evidence of pulmonary TB at chest radiography.
b. disease is typically bilateral.
c. renal calcification occurs in most cases.
d. cavities seen at IVU do not communicate with the collecting system.
e. tramline calcification of the vas deferens is characteristic.

18. Medullary nephrocalcinosis occurs in:

a. hypoparathyroidism.
b. renal tubular acidosis type IV.
c. milk–alkali syndrome.
d. hypervitaminosis D.
e. medullary sponge kidney.

19. Renal transitional cell carcinoma:

a. predominantly affects males.
b. is predisposed to by analgesic abuse.
c. is associated with synchronous tumour in 50–60%.
d. commonly spreads haematogenously.
e. is suggested by upper urinary tract calcification on a plain radiograph.

20. Regarding autosomal dominant polycystic kidney disease:

a. there is an association with mitral valve prolapse.
b. internal haemorrhage often occurs with extrarenal cysts.
c. there is an association with bicuspid aortic valve.
d. the commonest cause of death is subarachnoid haemorrhage.
e. associated calculi are commonly radiolucent.

21. Malakoplakia of the urinary tract:

a. is usually secondary to fungal infection.
b. is most common in the renal pelvis.
c. is associated with enlarged kidneys at CT.
d. is limited by the renal capsule.
e. may result in cholesteatoma of the collecting system.

22. Recognised findings in acute pyelonephritis include:

a. delayed pelvicalyceal filling at IVU.
b. a striated nephrogram.
c. reduced parenchymal reflectivity at US.
d. wedges of parenchymal low attenuation at enhanced CT.
e. areas of low signal at T2-weighted MRI.

23. **The following are true of CT:**

a. both the x-ray tube and detectors rotate in fourth generation scanners.
b. most scanners now use filtered back projection reconstruction.
c. gas-filled ionisation chambers are more sensitive detectors than scintillation crystals.
d. the Hounsfield number of water is independent of tube kV.
e. beam hardening software algorithms allow for less filtration to be used.

24. **Concerning pelvic ultrasound:**

a. a 12 MHz transducer is necessary for transvaginal US.
b. uterine tubes are often seen as linear structures of increased reflectivity at transabdominal US.
c. the cervix constitutes two-thirds of the length of the pre-pubertal uterus.
d. in the proliferative phase, an endometrial thickness of 7–12 mm is normal.
e. ovarian vessels communicate with the ovaries from the postero-lateral direction.

25. **Placental enlargement at US may be caused by:**

a. syphilis.
b. thalassaemia.
c. diabetes mellitus.
d. pre-eclampsia.
e. fetal chromosomal abnormalities.

26. **Concerning the gestation sac at US:**

a. a mean sac diameter of 5 mm corresponds to a gestational age of 5 weeks.
b. the sac normally lies within the uterine cavity.
c. two surrounding rings of reflectivity are specific for a pseudosac.
d. a 'chorionic rim' of increased reflectivity is seen around most sacs.
e. the smallest detectable sac has a mean diameter of 2–3 mm.

27. **Regarding fetal US:**

a. the choroid plexus is of low reflectivity.
b. the cardiac ventricle nearest the anterior chest wall is the left ventricle.
c. the yolk sac lies within the gestation sac.
d. the fourth ventricle is normally visible.
e. the thalamus is of high reflectivity.

28. The following are true of omphalocoele:

a. there is an association with bladder exstrophy.
b. the defect is usually right-sided.
c. maternal serum alpha-fetoprotein is elevated.
d. the herniated bowel is not covered by a membrane.
e. there is a low incidence of associated chromosomal abnormalities.

29. Concerning ectopic pregnancy:

a. it is a contraindication to transvaginal US.
b. the absence of free fluid at US virtually excludes the diagnosis.
c. an adnexal mass with a yolk sac is found at US in 15–20%.
d. the corpus luteum indicates the side of the pregnancy.
e. location in the cervix is a life-threatening event.

30. Concerning lutein cysts:

a. theca lutein cysts are usually unilateral.
b. theca lutein cysts typically contain internal echoes at transvaginal US.
c. corpus luteum cysts are associated with delayed menstruation.
d. corpus luteum cysts are painful.
e. corpus luteum cysts are associated with tamoxifen therapy.

31. The following are true of ovarian cancer:

a. CA-125 is elevated in 80–90% of FIGO stage I tumours.
b. the primary mode of spread is lymphatic.
c. most tumours have a stromal origin.
d. tumour rupture can lead to pseudomyxoma peritonei.
e. FIGO stage II tumours are confined to the pelvis.

32. Endometrial carcinoma:

a. is of lower signal than normal endometrium at T2-weighted MRI.
b. is a concern if the endometrial thickness is 7 mm in a post-menopausal woman.
c. is usually an adenocarcinoma.
d. is of lower signal than myometrium at T2-weighted MRI.
e. is more accurately staged by MRI with the use of IV Gd-DTPA.

33. **Adenomyosis:**

a. is seen as thickening of the junctional zone at T1-weighted MRI.
b. is visible at CT.
c. is commonly associated with endometriosis.
d. results in myometrial cysts at transvaginal US.
e. is a recognised cause of infertility.

34. **Carcinoma of the cervix:**

a. is of higher signal than normal cervix at T1-weighted MRI.
b. can mimic Nabothian cysts.
c. is a cause of a fluid-filled uterus.
d. is most often adenocarcinoma.
e. causes blurring of the uterine junctional zone at T2-weighted MRI.

35. **Concerning the anatomy of the female breast:**

a. the breast extends from the second to the ninth costal cartilage.
b. blood supply is from the internal and lateral thoracic arteries.
c. venous drainage occurs to the azygos vein.
d. lymphatic drainage is via the intercostal chains.
e. the level of the lymph nodes is defined by their relationship to the pectoralis major muscle.

36. **Hormone replacement therapy:**

a. causes enlargement of fibroadenomas.
b. with tibolone has the greatest effect on mammographic density.
c. reduces the specificity of screening mammography.
d. only reduces the sensitivity of screening mammography in women over 50.
e. used long-term increases the risk of breast cancer four-fold.

37. **Fibroadenomas:**

a. are well vascularised.
b. have a characteristic halo at US.
c. are typically heterogeneous on US.
d. produce edge shadowing.
e. can show calcification.

38. Regarding breast MRI:

a. cysts are of low signal at T1-weighting.
b. non-enhancing internal septations are a strong predictor of malignancy.
c. ductal carcinoma is typically low signal at both T1- and T2-weighting.
d. rim enhancement has a high predictive value for benignity.
e. centripetal enhancement has a high predictive value for malignancy.

39. Features of a lesion at breast US that suggest malignancy include:

a. increased reflectivity relative to fat.
b. AP diameter greater than transverse.
c. angular margins.
d. a thin, reflective capsule.
e. acoustic shadowing.

40. Ductal carcinoma in situ:

a. can present with Paget's disease of the nipple.
b. accounts for 15–20% of breast cancers at screening mammography.
c. detected at screening are usually low grade tumours.
d. showing linear branching calcification is usually a high grade tumour.
e. confers a 3–5% risk of developing invasive cancer within 10 years.

Module Four: Examination Two – Answers

1. Answers

a. **False** – stabilised microbubbles of air or perfluorocarbon.
b. **False** – at less than 10 μm, they pass through capillary beds.
c. **True**
d. **False** – some agents, e.g. Levovist, have a hepatosplenic-specific parenchymal phase after the blood-pool phase.
e. **False**

(Harvey CJ, Pilcher JM, Eckersley RJ et al. Advances in ultrasound. *Clin Radiol* 2002;57:157–177)

2. Answers

a. **False** – the membranous segment is the narrowest.
b. **True**
c. **True**
d. **False** – internal pudendal artery.
e. **True**

(Butler et al. p286)

3. Answers

a. **False** – posterolateral surface.
b. **False** – para-aortic nodes.
c. **False** – anterior to the artery.
d. **False** – it drains into the IVC.
e. **False** – it is a longitudinal structure, of high reflectivity at US.

(Ryan & McNicholas pp223–225)

4. Answers

a. **False** – DTPA is excreted by glomerular filtration.
b. **False** – it is excreted by tubular secretion, but allows measurement of effective renal plasma flow.
c. **True**
d. **True**
e. **True**

(Chapman & Nakielny 2001 pp166–169)

5. Answers

a. **False** – adrenal haemorrhage is the commonest cause.
b. **True** – enlarged adrenal glands with hepatosplenomegaly.
c. **True**
d. **True** – due to previous haemorrhage.
e. **True**

(Brant & Helms p774)

6. Answers

a. **False** – no malignant potential exists.
b. **False** – calcification is present in up to 20%.
c. **True** – usually larger than 10 cm.
d. **False** – they arise from haemopoietic elements.
e. **False** – they are frequently heterogeneous due to mixed internal components.

(Brant & Helms pp773–774)

7. Answers

a. **False** – most cases are 5 cm or larger.
b. **False** – the sympathetic chains and organ of Zuckerkandl are the usual site.
c. **True** – in 10%, also seen are necrosis and cystic change.
d. **True** – the risk of hypertensive crisis is small with low osmolar contrast.
e. **False** – it is isointense or of reduced signal at T1-weighting.

(Haaga et al. pp1520–1521)

8. Answers

a. **False** – most common in the elderly.
b. **True**
c. **False** – they appear avascular.
d. **False** – more common on the left.
e. **False** – thickened.

(Sutton pp1023–1024)

9. Answers

a. **False** – tumours are of lower signal than normal testis on T2-weighting.
b. **False**
c. **False** – they are not commonly involved.
d. **True**
e. **True**

(Brant & Helms p823)

10. Answers

a. **False** – the transitional zone hypertrophies.
b. **True**
c. **False** – no correlation.
d. **True**
e. **True** – characteristically periurethral.

(Sutton pp1004–1005)

11. Answers

a. **True**
b. **True**
c. **True**
d. **False** – T2-weighting, appears as foci of low signal.
e. **False**

(Grainger & Allison pp1639–1641; Dähnert p941; Haaga et al. pp1768–1772)

12. Answers

- **a. False** – *Schistosoma haematobium* is the usual causative agent.
- **b. False** – aperistaltic ureters.
- **c. True** – with irregular dilatation.
- **d. False** – the calcification is due to submucosal ova, and does not cause rigidity.
- **e. False** – renal disease develops slowly due to functional obstruction and reflux.

(Brant & Helms pp801–804; Grainger & Allison p1551)

13. Answers

- **a. True**
- **b. True**
- **c. False** – nine times more common in men.
- **d. True** – secondary to chronic inflammation.
- **e. False** – multiple in approximately half of cases.

(Dähnert pp913–914)

14. Answers

- **a. False** – emphysematous cystitis occurs almost exclusively in diabetes, cystitis cystica is characterised by multiple cystic mucosal elevations.
- **b. True** – if associated with emphysematous cystitis.
- **c. True**
- **d. True** – these fungal balls may be mobile, *Candida* is the usual cause.
- **e. False** – most common at the floor of the bladder.

(Grainger & Allison pp1618–1619; Dähnert pp916–917)

15. Answers

- **a. True**
- **b. True**
- **c. True**
- **d. True**
- **e. False** – bulbous urethra.

(Grainger & Allison pp1645–1648; Dähnert p979)

16. Answers

- **a. False** – in adults, underlying renal disease such as membranous glomerulonephritis is the commonest cause.
- **b. True**
- **c. True** – occasionally.
- **d. False** – there is persistence of corticomedullary differentiation.
- **e. False** – thrombus is low signal on gradient echo sequences.

(Grainger & Allison pp1523–1524)

17. Answers

a. **True**
b. **False** – usually unilateral, when bilateral it is asymmetrical.
c. **False** – 25–30%.
d. **False** – they communicate.
e. **False** – beaded calcification is the typical pattern, tramline calcification occurs in diabetes.

(Grainger & Allison pp1547–1549; Dähnert pp975–976)

18. Answers

a. **False** – hyperparathyroidism.
b. **False** – type I renal tubular acidosis.
c. **True**
d. **True**
e. **True**

(Brant & Helms pp789–790)

19. Answers

a. **True**
b. **True**
c. **False** – 25% have synchronous tumour.
d. **False** – it is rare, nodal spread is more common.
e. **False** – it virtually never calcifies.

(Sutton pp959–960)

20. Answers

a. **True**
b. **False** – it is rare.
c. **True**
d. **False** – renal failure is the commonest cause of mortality.
e. **True** – urinary calculi occur in 20–35% and are urate stones in over half.

(Brant & Helms pp783–785; Dähnert pp936–937)

21. Answers

a. **False** – secondary to chronic *E. coli* infection in middle-aged women.
b. **False** – most common in bladder, then lower and upper ureter, then renal pelvis.
c. **True**
d. **False**
e. **False** – cholesteatoma is secondary to leukoplakia.

(Grainger & Allison p1553; Dähnert p924; Haaga et al. p1586)

22. Answers

a. **True**
b. **True** – or an immediate dense nephrogram.
c. **True** – foci of increased reflectivity are also described.
d. **True** – which show enhancement at delayed imaging (3–6 hours).
e. **False** – high signal wedges.

(Grainger & Allison pp1543–1544; Dähnert pp942–943)

23. Answers

a. **False** – only the tube rotates in fourth generation machines.
b. **True** – allows for a short reconstruction time.
c. **False** – less sensitive, but more stable and have less lag.
d. **True** – it is zero by definition.
e. **True** – typically 3 mm Al in a modern scanner.

(Dendy & Heaton pp256–263; Farr & Allisy-Roberts pp100–109; Haaga et al. p15)

24. Answers

a. **False** – transducers are usually 7.5–10 MHz.
b. **False** – the uterine tubes are not usually visible at transabdominal US.
c. **True**
d. **False** – 4–6 mm is normal.
e. **True**

(Ryan & McNicholas pp225–231)

25. Answers

a. **True**
b. **True** – alpha-thalassaemia.
c. **True**
d. **False** – causes a small placenta.
e. **True** – may also cause a small placenta.

(Chapman & Nakielny 2003 pp513–514; Dähnert p991)

26. Answers

a. **True**
b. **False** – it lies within the endometrial layer.
c. **False** – the 'double decidua' sign is specific for a gestation sac, but is absent in one third.
d. **True** – 80%.
e. **True**

(Dewbury et al. vol. 3 pp155–156)

27. Answers

a. **False** – choroid plexus is of high reflectivity.
b. **False** – right ventricle.
c. **True**
d. **False**
e. **False** – low reflectivity.

(Brant & Helms pp881–883 & 915)

28. Answers

a. **True**
b. **False** – the defect is midline, it is usually right-sided in gastroschisis.
c. **True** – in up to 70% of cases.
d. **False** – there is an amniotic covering, in contradistinction to gastroschisis.
e. **False** – there is a high incidence of associated chromosomal abnormalities.

(Chapman & Nakielny 2003 p505)

29. Answers

a. **False**
b. **False**
c. **True**
d. **False** – one third implant in the contralateral tube.
e. **True**

(Dewbury et al. vol. 3 pp178–181)

30. Answers

a. **False** – usually bilateral.
b. **False** – when haemorrhagic they contain internal echoes.
c. **True**
d. **True**
e. **False**

(Grainger & Allison p2215; Dähnert pp1048–1049)

31. Answers

a. **False** – elevated in 25–50%.
b. **False** – peritoneal seeding is more common.
c. **False** – 60–70% are epithelial tumours.
d. **True**
e. **True**

(Brant & Helms pp817–818)

32. Answers

a. **True**
b. **True** – any thickness over 5 mm is suspicious.
c. **True**
d. **False** – hyperintense to myometrium.
e. **True**

(Dähnert p1032)

33. Answers

a. **False** – seen at T2-weighted MRI.
b. **False**
c. **False** – endometriosis is associated in 35–40%.
d. **True**
e. **True**

(Dähnert p1022)

34. Answers

a. **False** – it is the same signal on T1-weighting, and hyperintense on T2.
b. **True**
c. **True**
d. **False** – 95% are squamous carcinomas.
e. **True** – also widening, due to retained secretions secondary to obstruction of the os.

(Dähnert pp1024–1025)

35. Answers

a. **False** – second to sixth costal cartilages.
b. **True**
c. **True**
d. **True**
e. **False** – defined by relationship to pectoralis minor.

(Butler et al. p174)

36. Answers

a. **True** – also enlargement of cysts, and increase in breast density.
b. **False** – tibolone has little, if any effect.
c. **True** – by 12–50%, mainly at incident screens.
d. **True** – by 7–21%.
e. **False** – the Million Women Study found that the relative risk is 2.0 for combined preparations, and 1.3 for progestogen-only HRT.

(Evans A. Hormone replacement therapy and mammographic screening. *Clin Radiol* 2002;57:563–564)

37. Answers

a. **False** – they are poorly vascular.
b. **False** – no halo.
c. **False** – they appear homogeneous.
d. **True**
e. **True**

(Dewbury et al. p777)

38. Answers

a. **True**
b. **False** – a predictor of benignity.
c. **True**
d. **False** – predictive of malignancy.
e. **True**

(Sutton p1477)

39. Answers

a. **True** – but less reflective than surrounding fibrous tissue.
b. **True**
c. **True**
d. **False**
e. **True**

(Dähnert pp539–540)

40. Answers

- a. **True** – also with a palpable mass, or nipple discharge.
- b. **True** – and 3–5% of clinically-detected cancers.
- c. **False** – 80% of screening-detected DCIS is high grade.
- d. **True** – this appearance has a high predictive value.
- e. **False** – 30–50% risk of invasive cancer.

(Kessar P, Perry N, Vinnicombe SJ et al. How significant is detection of ductal carcinoma in situ in a breast screening programme? *Clin Radiol* 2002;57:807–814)

Module Four: Examination Three – Questions

1. **The following are true concerning the bioeffects of MRI:**

   a. the main static field can cause ECG changes.
   b. MRI is contraindicated in the first trimester of pregnancy.
   c. gradient fields can cause visual disturbances.
   d. the cornea is the part of the body most susceptible to heating from RF pulses.
   e. tattoos can heat up during scanning.

2. **The following are true of renal anatomy:**

   a. the upper poles lie anterior to the lower poles.
   b. the anterior pararenal space is confined laterally by the lateroconal fascia.
   c. the right renal vein receives the gonadal vein in 5–10%.
   d. the glomeruli develop from the metanephron.
   e. pelvic kidneys are usually supplied by a branch of the external iliac artery.

3. **Prophylactic antibiotics are indicated for:**

   a. percutaneous nephrostomy.
   b. percutaneous nephrolithotomy.
   c. micturating cystourethrography in adults.
   d. ascending urethrography.
   e. transrectal prostate biopsy.

4. **Regarding contrast media:**

   a. iopromide is a non-ionic dimer.
   b. osmolality depends on the size of the contrast molecule.
   c. salivary gland swelling can follow intravascular administration.
   d. high osmolar contrast media inhibit thrombin formation.
   e. sodium salts produce less diuresis than meglumine salts at IVU.

5. **Adrenal carcinoma:**

   a. is associated with astrocytoma.
   b. is hyperintense to the liver at T2-weighted MRI.
   c. results in enlarged adrenal arteries at angiography.
   d. is commonly calcified at CT.
   e. rarely metastasizes to the liver.

6. **The following adrenal lesions lose signal at opposed-phase MRI.**

   a. myelolipoma.
   b. adrenal carcinoma.
   c. phaeochromocytoma.
   d. metastatic melanoma.
   e. Conn's tumour.

7. **Non-functioning adrenal cortical adenomas:**

   a. are usually larger than 5 cm when detected.
   b. frequently have attenuations of 10 HU or less at unenhanced CT.
   c. do not enhance at CT following IV contrast.
   d. following IV Gd-DTPA, show rapid washout of enhancement at MRI.
   e. do not lose signal at opposed-phase MRI.

8. **Seminoma:**

   a. is the commonest tumour of the testis.
   b. typically causes elevated serum alpha-fetoprotein.
   c. often replaces the entire testis with tumour.
   d. extends to the epididymis in 30–50%.
   e. is of lower signal than normal testis at T2-weighted MRI.

9. **Testicular microlithiasis:**

   a. characteristically causes acoustic shadowing on ultrasound.
   b. is unilateral in half of cases.
   c. is seen in 1–5% of men referred for scrotal ultrasound.
   d. is associated with testicular germ cell neoplasia.
   e. occurs as a response to treatment for lymphoma.

10. **Regarding benign prostatic hypertrophy:**

    a. the urethra appears shortened at MCUG.
    b. the ureters may show 'fish-hook' deformity at IVU.
    c. mixed reflectivity of the central gland at transrectal US is characteristic.
    d. distinction from prostate cancer is not possible at T2-weighted MRI.
    e. outflow obstruction is excluded by complete bladder emptying at US.

11. **Regarding MRI of the post-radiotherapy bladder:**

a. radiation injury occurs in 60–80%.
b. the mucosa is of high signal at T1-weighting in the acute stage.
c. the outer wall returns high signal at T2-weighting in the long term.
d. signal changes initially occur around the bladder neck.
e. haematuria is a long-term complication.

12. **Involvement of the urinary bladder by tuberculosis:**

a. usually arises from a renal source.
b. causes thickening of the bladder wall at US.
c. commonly results in bladder wall calcification.
d. results in a diminished bladder capacity.
e. causes filling defects at cystography.

13. **Urethral carcinoma:**

a. is more common in men.
b. is associated with previous trauma.
c. of the proximal urethra presents early.
d. is of low signal intensity at T1-weighted MRI.
e. has nodal metastases in most cases at presentation.

14. **Concerning US of the transplant kidney:**

a. it is not possible to differentiate acute tubular necrosis and acute rejection.
b. acute rejection causes increased pyramidal reflectivity.
c. absence of diastolic arterial flow is usually due to acute tubular necrosis.
d. absence of intrarenal flow at colour Doppler is pathognomonic of arterial thrombosis.
e. reversed diastolic arterial flow occurs with venous thrombosis.

15. **Causes of a unilateral enlarged kidney include:**

a. obstructive uropathy.
b. radiation nephritis.
c. renal artery stenosis.
d. acute renal vein thrombosis.
e. acute renal infarction.

16. **The following are associated with von Hippel–Lindau disease:**

a. multiple pancreatic cysts.
b. renal adenomas.
c. cerebellar hamartomas.
d. retinal angiomas.
e. renal cell carcinoma, which is frequently multicentric.

17. **Regarding renal papillary necrosis:**

a. focal cortical loss between the calyces is typical.
b. when associated with infection, it is usually unilateral.
c. there is an association with squamous cell carcinoma.
d. the septa of Bertin enlarge.
e. the lower pole calyces are characteristically affected first.

18. **Emphysematous pyelonephritis:**

a. occurs almost exclusively in diabetics.
b. may be caused by *Candida albicans*.
c. is bilateral in fewer than 10%.
d. has a worse prognosis if associated with a renal fluid collection at CT.
e. is a contraindication to CT-guided drainage.

19. **Renal cell carcinoma:**

a. shows calcification on abdominal radiographs in 20–35%.
b. when small, is usually of increased reflectivity at US.
c. appears hypervascular at corticomedullary phase contrast-enhanced CT.
d. returns heterogeneous low signal at T1-weighted MRI.
e. metastases to bone are typically osteolytic.

20. **The following are true concerning renal lymphoma:**

a. it is secondary to lymphoma elsewhere in 30–50%.
b. disease is usually bilateral.
c. diffuse infiltration is the commonest appearance at CT.
d. the renal vein usually remains patent despite tumour encasement.
e. lymphoma enhances less than normal cortex at MRI following IV Gd-DTPA.

21. Pelviureteric junction obstruction:

a. is associated with an accessory renal artery in 20%.
b. is bilateral in 5%.
c. is associated with multicystic disease of the kidney.
d. the ureter distal to the obstruction is usually atretic.
e. is associated with stone formation.

22. Lateral deviation of the ureters at IVU may be due to:

a. pelvic lipomatosis.
b. retrocaval ureter.
c. para-aortic lymphadenopathy.
d. abdominoperineal resection.
e. ovarian dermoid.

23. Tissue harmonic imaging in US:

a. uses a low transmit frequency.
b. forms the image from the second harmonic signal.
c. has a worse signal-to-noise ratio than conventional grey-scale US.
d. improves detection of gallstones.
e. depends upon the linear propagation of sound through tissues.

24. Regarding the female genital tract:

a. a retroverted uterus indents the anterior rectal wall.
b. the uterus has no peritoneal covering.
c. the uterine tubes are 10–12 cm long.
d. the cervical canal shortens after childbirth.
e. the cervix drains to the internal and external iliac nodes.

25. The following are associated with polyhydramnios:

a. maternal diabetes mellitus.
b. duodenal atresia.
c. trisomy 13.
d. ventricular septal defect.
e. cystic adenomatoid lung.

26. 'Soft' markers of chromosomal abnormality at antenatal US include:

a. choroid plexus cysts.
b. foci of increased reflectivity in the cardiac ventricles.
c. increased reflectivity of bowel.
d. a single umbilical artery.
e. cystic hygroma.

27. **Nuchal thickness is increased in:**
    a. trisomy 18.
    b. congenital diaphragmatic hernia.
    c. Pierre Robin syndrome.
    d. fetal hydrops.
    e. fragile X syndrome.

28. **Causes of fetal ascites include:**
    a. rhesus incompatibility.
    b. twin-to-twin transfusion syndrome.
    c. Turner's syndrome.
    d. toxoplasmosis.
    e. congenital diaphragmatic hernia.

29. **Regarding polycystic ovary syndrome:**
    a. the endometrium appears thinned at transvaginal US.
    b. the typical US appearances are seen in 20% of normal women.
    c. ovarian stroma is usually of increased reflectivity at US.
    d. ovarian volume is related to the degree of hormonal disturbance.
    e. the cysts are characteristically central in location.

30. **In the staging and follow-up of ovarian cancer:**
    a. ascites is not a feature of stage I disease.
    b. prognosis is independent of histological subtype.
    c. CA-125 is elevated by endometriosis.
    d. omental cake is a common feature of recurrent disease.
    e. peritoneal deposits enhance at MRI following IV Gd-DTPA.

31. **MRI features of uterine leiomyomas include:**
    a. clear margination from the surrounding myometrium.
    b. a high signal pseudocapsule at T2-weighting.
    c. heterogeneous high signal at T2-weighting in most cases.
    d. increased signal intensity at T2-weighting following myxoid degeneration.
    e. no enhancement following IV Gd-DTPA.

32. **Endometrial carcinoma:**
    a. is present in 50% of women with endometrial thickness greater than 15 mm.
    b. is associated with high resistance waveforms at Doppler US.
    c. cannot be distinguished from adenomyosis at MRI.
    d. has usually extended beyond the uterus at presentation.
    e. is associated with endometrioid ovarian carcinoma.

33. **CT features of pelvic inflammatory disease include:**

a. thickening of the uterosacral ligaments.
b. enlarged, polycystic ovaries.
c. an enlarged, heterogeneously enhancing cervix.
d. hydronephrosis.
e. tubo-ovarian abscess, usually containing gas.

34. **Ovarian vein thrombosis:**

a. occurs in pelvic inflammatory disease.
b. is most common on the right.
c. is not associated with pulmonary embolism.
d. complicates cytoreductive surgery for ovarian cancer.
e. is best diagnosed by Doppler US.

35. **Regarding the use of ultrasound in breast imaging:**

a. a high frequency probe should be used.
b. microcalcifications can be identified because of their acoustic shadowing.
c. tissue harmonic imaging is unhelpful.
d. compression should always be used.
e. the nipple is highly attenuating.

36. **The NHS Breast Screening Programme:**

a. is only open to women aged 50 to 70 years.
b. requires double-reading of all mammograms.
c. detects 13 cancers per 1000 women screened.
d. uses two-view mammography for all screening rounds.
e. invites women to attend at two-yearly intervals.

37. **Indications for mammography include:**

a. screening of asymptomatic women over the age of 50 years.
b. symptomatic breast lumps in a woman aged 30 years.
c. as a baseline prior to commencing hormone replacement therapy.
d. inflammatory diseases of the breast.
e. surveillance following local excision of tumour.

38. **Cystosarcoma phylloides:**

a. grows rapidly.
b. is most common in women aged 20–30 years.
c. shows florid calcification at mammography.
d. is usually benign.
e. undergoes degeneration into osteosarcoma.

39. Fat necrosis of the breast:

a. occurs after 15–40% of breast biopsies.
b. is exquisitely tender.
c. causes skin retraction.
d. results in a spiculated mass at mammography.
e. causes acoustic shadowing at US.

40. Concerning carcinoma of the breast:

a. a spiculated mass is the commonest mammographic appearance.
b. microcalcification is present in 65% of DCIS.
c. invasive ductal carcinoma accounts for approximately 95%.
d. the upper outer quadrant is the commonest site.
e. retroareolar carcinoma is uncommon.

Module Four: Examination Three – Answers

1. Answers

a. **True** – increase in height of T-waves.
b. **False** – but it should be avoided, where possible.
c. **True** – magnetophosphenes occur due to a time-varying magnetic field.
d. **True**
e. **True**

(Westbrook & Kaut pp235–238)

2. Answers

a. **False** – the lower poles are more anterior.
b. **True**
c. **True**
d. **False** – from the mesonephron.
e. **False** – arterial supply is usually from the internal iliac artery.

(Brant & Helms pp776–777; Ryan & McNicholas pp184–189)

3. Answers

a. **True**
b. **True**
c. **False**
d. **True**
e. **True**

(Chapman & Nakielny 2001 pp141–160)

4. Answers

a. **False** – it is a non-ionic monomer.
b. **False** – it depends on the number of particles in solution.
c. **True**
d. **True** – low osmolar contrast does not have this anticoagulant effect.
e. **True**

(Grainger & Allison pp29–39)

5. Answers

a. **True**
b. **True**
c. **True**
d. **False** – calcification is seen in 30%.
e. **False** – liver metastases are common.

(Brant & Helms pp771–772)

6. Answers

a. **True** – due to the fat content.
b. **False**
c. **False**
d. **False**
e. **True**

(Haaga et al. pp1514–1529)

7. Answers

a. **False** – most are less than 3 cm.
b. **True**
c. **False** – they show rapid early enhancement, with more than 60% washout at delayed CT.
d. **True**
e. **False**

(Haaga et al. pp1523–1525; Dähnert p910)

8. Answers

a. **True** – patients are usually in the fourth or fifth decade of life.
b. **False** – beta-hCG is elevated, alpha-fetoprotein is not elevated in pure seminoma.
c. **True** – in over 50%.
d. **False** – it is usually confined by the tunica albuginea.
e. **True**

(Dogra VS, Gottlieb RH, Oka M et al. Sonography of the scrotum. *Radiology* 2003;227:18–36)

9. Answers

a. **False** – shadowing is not observed in most cases.
b. **False** – unilateral in between 2.7% and 27%.
c. **True**
d. **True** – the nature of the relationship is contentious, however.
e. **False**

(Miller FNAC, Sidhu P. Does testicular microlithiasis matter? A review. *Clin Radiol* 2002;57:883–890)

10. Answers

a. **False** – narrowed and elongated.
b. **True**
c. **False** – both low and high reflectivity patterns are also well-recognised.
d. **True**
e. **False**

(Grainger & Allison pp1635–1636)

11. Answers

a. **False** – it occurs in 20%.
b. **True** – also high signal at T2-weighting, due to haemorrhagic oedema.
c. **True**
d. **False** – initially the changes are around the trigone and posterior wall.
e. **True** – due to telangiectasia.

(Husband & Reznek pp987–989)

12. Answers

- a. **True**
- b. **True** – also trabeculation.
- c. **False** – calcification occurs infrequently.
- d. **True** – due to scarring.
- e. **True** – caused by granulomas.

(Grainger & Allison p1619; Dähnert p976)

13. Answers

- a. **False** – twice as common in women.
- b. **True** – also associated with infection and urethral caruncles.
- c. **False** – presents late.
- d. **True** – at T2-weighting, carcinoma is of increased signal in men and decreased signal in women.
- e. **False** – lymphadenopathy is present in up to one third.

(Grainger & Allison pp1648–1650)

14. Answers

- a. **True**
- b. **True** – also decreased pyramidal reflectivity, increased corticomedullary differentiation, reduced renal sinus echoes.
- c. **False** – usually due to acute rejection.
- d. **False** – also seen in renal vein thrombosis and hyperacute rejection.
- e. **True** – a 'reverse M' pattern is characteristic.

(Baxter GM. Ultrasound of renal transplantation. *Clin Radiol* 2001;56:802–818)

15. Answers

- a. **True**
- b. **False** – small kidney.
- c. **False** – small kidney.
- d. **True**
- e. **True**

(Brant & Helms p789)

16. Answers

- a. **True**
- b. **True**
- c. **False** – cerebellar haemangioblastomas.
- d. **True**
- e. **True** – renal cell carcinoma is usually bilateral and multicentric.

(Brant & Helms p783)

17. Answers

a. **False** – cortical loss is unusual, and when present occurs over the calyces.
b. **True**
c. **True** – also with transitional cell carcinoma.
d. **True** – secondary to oedema.
e. **False** – although initially patchy, no particular pattern is described.

(Grainger & Allison pp1544–1547; Dähnert pp934–935)

18. Answers

a. **True** – 85–95% of cases occur in diabetics.
b. **True** – also *E. coli*, *Klebsiella*, *Proteus* and *Pseudomonas*.
c. **True**
d. **False** – associated with bubbly, loculated gas, this implies an effective immune response and is associated with an 18% mortality, versus 69% for lack of collections and streaky/mottled gas.
e. **False** – treatment is largely with antibiotics and nephrectomy, but there is a role for guided drainage.

(Grainger & Allison p1552; Dähnert p944; Haaga et al. p1584)

19. Answers

a. **False** – 30% show calcification at CT, but only 5–10% on plain films.
b. **True** – the appearance can mimic an angiomyolipoma.
c. **False** – tumour enhances to a lesser degree than normal kidney.
d. **True** – heterogeneous increased signal on T2-weighting.
e. **True** – and expansile.

(Grainger & Allison p1567; Dähnert pp950–952; Haaga et al. pp1559–1560)

20. Answers

a. **False** – primary lymphoma is extremely rare as the kidney contains no lymphoid tissue.
b. **True** – in 75%.
c. **False** – multiple low attenuation nodules are the commonest pattern.
d. **True** – a characteristic finding.
e. **True**

(Grainger & Allison p1572; Haaga et al. pp1570–1571)

21. Answers

a. **True**
b. **False** – 20%.
c. **True**
d. **False** – usually normal.
e. **True**

(Sutton pp938–940)

22. Answers

a. **False** – medial deviation.
b. **False** – causes medial deviation of the right ureter only.
c. **True**
d. **False** – causes medial deviation.
e. **True**

(Dähnert p886)

23. Answers

a. **True**
b. **True**
c. **False** – better signal-to-noise and contrast resolution.
d. **True** – also better characterisation of cystic lesions.
e. **False** – relies on non-linear propagation.

(Harvey CJ, Pilcher JM, Eckersley RJ et al. Advances in ultrasound. *Clin Radiol* 2002;57:157–177)

24. Answers

a. **True**
b. **False**
c. **True**
d. **True**
e. **True**

(Ryan & McNicholas pp225–230; Brant & Helms p815)

25. Answers

a. **True**
b. **True**
c. **True**
d. **True**
e. **True**

(Dähnert pp989–990)

26. Answers

a. **True** – also mild ventriculomegaly.
b. **True**
c. **True** – also dilatation of the renal pelvis.
d. **False** – this is a 'hard' marker.
e. **False** – this is strongly associated with chromosomal abnormalities.

(Chapman & Nakielny 2003 p503)

27. Answers

a. **True** – also trisomy 21 and other aneuploidies.
b. **True** – also multicystic dysplastic kidney and cystic hygroma.
c. **True** – also Noonan syndrome.
d. **True**
e. **False**

(Dewbury et al. vol. 3 pp285–286)

28. Answers

a. **True**
b. **True**
c. **True**
d. **True**
e. **True**

(Chapman & Nakielny 2003 p500)

29. Answers

a. **False** – it appears thickened.
b. **True**
c. **True** – in most cases.
d. **False**
e. **False** – peripheral.

(Sutton p1072; Dähnert p1057; Bates pp99–100)

30. Answers

a. **False** – ascites is a feature of FIGO stage Ic.
b. **True** – clinical (FIGO) staging is more relevant.
c. **True**
d. **False** – the greater omentum is usually removed at cytoreductive surgery.
e. **True**

(Haaga et al. p1792 & pp1734–1738)

31. Answers

a. **True**
b. **True** – in one third.
c. **False** – fibroids are usually of low signal at T2-weighting.
d. **True**
e. **False** – variable patterns of enhancement are seen.

(Grainger & Allison p2209; Dähnert p1063; Haaga et al. p1777)

32. Answers

a. **True** – compared to 10% with endometrium of 6–15 mm.
b. **False** – low resistance waveform, with RI < 0.7.
c. **False**
d. **False** – 75% of cases are FIGO stage I at presentation.
e. **True**

(Grainger & Allison pp2211–2212; Dähnert p1032; Haaga et al. p1731)

33. Answers

a. **True** – along with obscuration of pelvic fascial planes, this is an early finding.
b. **True** – abnormally enhancing, with stranding of surrounding fat.
c. **True**
d. **True** – due to functional or mechanical ureteric obstruction.
e. **False** – tubo-ovarian abscesses only occasionally contain gas.

(Sam JW, Jacobs JE, Birnbaum BA. Spectrum of CT findings in acute pyogenic pelvic inflammatory disease. *Radiographics* 2002;22:1327–1334)

34. Answers

a. **True**
b. **True**
c. **False** – 25% cases are associated with PE.
d. **True**
e. **False** – contrast-enhanced CT is superior.

(Dähnert p1050)

35. Answers

a. **True**
b. **False** – they can be seen but do not shadow.
c. **False** – harmonics are helpful by improving contrast and reducing artefact.
d. **False** – compression should be avoided when using Doppler.
e. **True**

(Dewbury et al. pp753–759)

36. Answers

a. **False** – women aged 50–70 are invited to attend, women over 70 are encouraged to self-refer.
b. **False** – although most units (76%) do double-read.
c. **False** – the NHSBSP detects approximately 6 cancers per 1000 women screened.
d. **True** – CC and MLO views at each attendance have been standard since 2003.
e. **False** – women attend every three years.

(Grainger & Allison pp2277–2280)

37. Answers

a. **True**
b. **False** – this is an indication for US.
c. **False** – not an indication.
d. **False** – indication for US.
e. **True**

(The Royal College of Radiologists. *Guidance on screening and symptomatic breast imaging.* 2nd edn. 2003; Sutton p1456)

38. Answers

a. **True** – may fill entire breast.
b. **False** – usually 40–50 years.
c. **False** – large, smooth, non-calcified mass
d. **True**
e. **True** – or liposarcoma/fibrosarcoma/histiosarcoma/chondrosarcoma.

(Dähnert p557)

39. Answers

a. **False** – 0.5% of biopsies.
b. **False** – usually clinically occult.
c. **True** – and skin thickening, in some cases.
d. **True** – may be indistinguishable from cancer.
e. **True** – especially if calcification is present.

(Dähnert pp557–558)

40. Answers

a. **True**
b. **False** – 95%.
c. **True**
d. **True**
e. **False** – second commonest location.

(Grainger & Allison p2251)

MODULE FIVE

Paediatrics

Time Allowed: 1 hour

Module Five: Examination One – Questions

1. **Technetium-99m is considered a good isotope for radionuclide imaging studies because:**

   a. it emits near monoenergetic gamma rays.
   b. it decays by electron capture.
   c. it has a half life of 6 hours.
   d. it decays to a daughter with a long half life.
   e. it is readily available from a generator.

2. **With respect to development of the skeleton:**

   a. the distal femoral epiphysis is ossified at birth.
   b. the calcaneal apophysis is normally denser than the calcaneum.
   c. the scapula ossifies in membrane.
   d. the posterior vertebral arches fuse in a craniocaudal direction.
   e. the os vesalianum pedis lies on the dorsum of the foot.

3. **When reducing an intussusception:**

   a. control of intraluminal pressure is better with barium than air.
   b. antibiotic cover is mandatory.
   c. dissection of air between the two layers heralds imminent reduction.
   d. fluid between intussusceptum and intussuscipiens predicts successful US reduction.
   e. pressure must not exceed 90 mmHg at air reduction.

4. **Congenital diaphragmatic hernias in liveborn infants:**

   a. are usually right-sided.
   b. do not contain retroperitoneal structures.
   c. are commonly associated with other congenital abnormalities.
   d. are associated with pulmonary hypoplasia.
   e. have a worse prognosis with an intra-thoracic stomach.

5. **Meconium aspiration syndrome:**

   a. is the commonest cause of respiratory distress in premature infants.
   b. is associated with placental insufficiency.
   c. results in air trapping on the chest radiograph.
   d. causes prominent air bronchograms.
   e. is associated with pneumothorax.

6. **Features of Ebstein's anomaly include:**

   a. tricuspid regurgitation.
   b. synchronous contraction of the proximal right ventricle with the right atrium.
   c. right atrial enlargement.
   d. pulmonary oligaemia.
   e. widened superior mediastinum.

7. **Regarding developmental dysplasia of the hip:**

   a. ultrasound assessment is practical up to 18 months of age.
   b. avascular necrosis is rare in untreated cases.
   c. an alpha angle of less than 50 degrees confirms a normal hip.
   d. it is more common on the right side.
   e. most dislocations occur during birth.

8. **If the bone age is greater than the chronological age, the following conditions should be considered:**

   a. polyostotic fibrous dysplasia.
   b. Cushing's syndrome.
   c. pseudohypoparathyroidism.
   d. hypothyroidism.
   e. coeliac disease.

9. **With respect to visceral injuries in non-accidental injury:**

   a. the liver is injured more commonly than the spleen.
   b. adrenal haemorrhage is more common on the left.
   c. duodenal haematoma has a 'coiled spring' appearance at contrast studies.
   d. intussusception is a recognised complication.
   e. the stomach is the most frequently ruptured part of the GI tract.

10. **In patients with Hirschsprung's disease:**

    a. skip lesions occur.
    b. a short segment of colon is affected in most cases.
    c. total colonic involvement is more common in males.
    d. there is an association with neuroblastoma.
    e. there is inversion of the rectosigmoid index.

11. In the diagnosis of infantile hypertrophic pyloric stenosis:

a. a palpable abdominal 'olive' is an indication for US.
b. contrast studies show reduced gastric peristalsis.
c. the pyloric canal is elongated at US.
d. a muscle wall thickness of 4 mm is a normal finding.
e. prolonged US scanning distinguishes pylorospasm from pyloric stenosis.

12. The following are true of tracheo-oesophageal fistula:

a. there is associated oesophageal atresia in 40–60%.
b. the atretic segment is usually in the distal third of the oesophagus.
c. a gasless abdomen at radiography indicates an H-type fistula.
d. further congenital anomalies are present in half of cases.
e. the diagnosis is suggested antenatally by polyhydramnios.

13. Posterior urethral valves:

a. are associated with pulmonary hypoplasia.
b. are associated with bladder neck hypertrophy.
c. usually form a horizontal web below the verumontanum.
d. are associated with vesicoureteric reflux at MCUG.
e. are obscured by an indwelling 6 F feeding tube for MCUG.

14. The following occur in prune belly syndrome:

a. bilateral cryptorchidism.
b. large kidneys.
c. narrowing of the bladder neck.
d. increased incidence of respiratory tract infections.
e. ureteric dilatation which is more marked distally.

15. Regarding horseshoe kidneys:

a. renal calculi are a recognised complication.
b. the superior mesenteric artery inhibits their normal ascent.
c. each moiety is commonly supplied by a single renal artery.
d. adrenal agenesis is a common accompaniment.
e. upper pole fusion occurs in 10–15% of cases.

16. Choanal atresia:

a. is due to a fibrous septum in the majority.
b. is most often bilateral.
c. causes lateral bowing of the lateral walls of the nasal cavity.
d. is associated with absence of the vomer at CT.
e. presents with respiratory distress.

17. **Radiological features of Arnold–Chiari malformations include:**

a. large foramen magnum.
b. convexity of the clivus.
c. hydrocephalus.
d. posterior displacement of the basilar artery.
e. absence of the septum pellucidum anteriorly.

18. **Retinoblastoma:**

a. is calcified at CT in most cases.
b. showing contrast enhancement at CT has a more favourable prognosis.
c. frequently extends extra-ocularly.
d. is usually bilateral.
e. is of high signal at T2-weighted MRI.

19. **Radiological features of achondroplasia include:**

a. wide foramen magnum.
b. champagne glass appearance of the pelvis.
c. an increase in lumbar vertebral interpedicular distance caudally.
d. notched growth plates.
e. short, narrow sciatic notches.

20. **The following are seen in patients with Turner's syndrome:**

a. scoliosis.
b. osteoporosis.
c. long fourth metacarpal.
d. carpal fusion.
e. coarctation of the aorta.

Module Five: Examination One – Answers

1. Answers

a. **True** – at 140 keV.
b. **False** – it decays by isomeric transition: $^{99m}Tc \rightarrow {}^{99}Tc$
c. **True**
d. **True** – the half life of ^{99}Tc is 2×10^5 years.
e. **True**

(Dendy & Heaton p190; Farr & Allisy-Roberts pp143–144)

2. Answers

a. **True**
b. **True**
c. **False** – the clavicle ossifies in membrane, the scapula ossifies in cartilage.
d. **False** – caudocranial, beginning in the lumbar region.
e. **False** – it lies proximal to the base of the fifth metatarsal.

(Butler et al. pp311, 332, 361, 375)

3. Answers

a. **False** – pressure is more accurately controlled with air reduction.
b. **False**
c. **False** – it means reduction is less likely.
d. **False** – trapped peritoneal fluid indicates likely failure of reduction.
e. **False** – up to 120 mmHg can be used for three minutes.

(Chapman & Nakielny 2001 pp75–78)

4. Answers

a. **False** – mostly occur on the left.
b. **False** – can rarely contain kidney, pancreas or adrenal.
c. **False** – only 20% in liveborn babies, compared to 90% in stillbirths.
d. **True**
e. **True**

(Dähnert pp482–483)

5. Answers

a. **False** – commonest cause in term/post-term babies.
b. **True**
c. **True**
d. **False** – not a feature.
e. **True** – in 25–40%.

(Grainger & Allison p638; Dähnert p504)

6. Answers

a. **True** – due to redundancy of the septal and posterior valve cusps.
b. **False** – although 'atrialised', the proximal RV contracts with the rest of the RV.
c. **True**
d. **True** – usually.
e. **False** – the vascular pedicle is narrow.

(Grainger & Allison pp811–812; Dähnert p627)

7. Answers

a. **False** – 8–10 months.
b. **False** – common.
c. **False** – an alpha angle of greater than 60 degrees indicates a normal hip.
d. **False** – more common on the left.
e. **False** – usually occur after birth.

(Dähnert pp63–66)

8. Answers

a. **True** – McCune–Albright syndrome, with precocious puberty.
b. **True** – also a cause of delayed bone age.
c. **True**
d. **False** – causes delayed bone age.
e. **False** – bone age is delayed.

(Reeder pp256–257)

9. Answers

a. **True**
b. **False** – more common on the right.
c. **True**
d. **True** – haematoma can act as a lead point.
e. **False** – more common at duodenojejunal flexure, and ileocaecal junction.

(Grainger & Allison pp2119–2122)

10. Answers

a. **True**
b. **True**
c. **False** – equal preponderance.
d. **True**
e. **True**

(Sutton pp860–861)

11. Answers

a. **False** – if the pylorus is palpable in the appropriate clinical setting, the diagnosis is established and imaging is not necessary.
b. **False** – increased peristalsis, which stops promptly at the pyloric antrum.
c. **True**
d. **False** – this is indicative of pyloric stenosis.
e. **True** – relaxation will eventually occur with pylorospasm.

(Hernanz-Schulman M. Infantile hypertrophic pyloric stenosis. *Radiology* 2003;227:319–331)

12. Answers

a. **False** – oesophageal atresia coexists with TOF in 90%.
b. **False** – atresia usually occurs at the junction of the proximal and middle third.
c. **False** – there is gas in the abdomen with an H-type fistula.
d. **True**
e. **True**

(Grainger & Allison pp1200–1201; Dähnert pp806–807)

13. Answers

a. **True** – due to oligohydramnios.
b. **True**
c. **False** – valves are most often mucosal folds, which extend inferiorly from the verumontanum.
d. **True** – in one third of cases.
e. **False** – the feeding tube need not be removed.

(Grainger & Allison pp1736–1738; Dähnert pp938–939)

14. Answers

a. **True**
b. **False** – small kidneys are seen.
c. **False** – the bladder neck is widened.
d. **True**
e. **True**

(Grainger & Allison pp1734–1735; Dähnert pp941–942)

15. Answers

a. **True**
b. **False** – inferior mesenteric artery.
c. **False** – renal arteries are usually multiple and ectopic in origin.
d. **False**
e. **True**

(Dähnert p920)

16. Answers

a. **False** – 85–90% are bony.
b. **True** – 60% are bilateral.
c. **False** – medial bowing.
d. **False** – thickening of the vomer.
e. **True** – neonates are obligate nose-breathers.

(Dähnert p375; Grainger & Allison p2616)

17. Answers

a. **True**
b. **False** – concavity.
c. **True**
d. **False** – anterior.
e. **True**

(Dähnert pp268–270)

18. Answers

a. **True**
b. **False** – is a poor prognostic sign.
c. **False** – occurs in 25% of cases.
d. **False** – 60% of cases are unilateral.
e. **False** – lower signal than the vitreous.

(Dähnert pp345–346)

19. Answers

a. **False** – narrow.
b. **True**
c. **False** – lack of or decrease.
d. **True**
e. **True**

(Dähnert p40)

20. Answers

a. **True**
b. **True**
c. **False** – short.
d. **True**
e. **True**

(Dähnert pp170–171)

Module Five: Examination Two – Questions

1. **Regarding the components of a modern US system:**
   a. time gain compensation reduces electronic noise in the received signal.
   b. radiofrequency (RF) oscillations in the received signal are removed by the RF amplifier.
   c. an 8-bit analogue-to-digital converter produces 4096 different digital numbers from the RF signal.
   d. reject control discards echoes below a certain amplitude.
   e. pre-processing curves are usually linear.

2. **The normal thymus in a child:**
   a. can lie inferior to the brachiocephalic artery.
   b. can extend into the posterior mediastinum.
   c. has a larger right lobe than left.
   d. can have a concave lateral margin.
   e. enhances following IV contrast.

3. **In the investigation of the paediatric urinary tract with radionuclide techniques:**
   a. ^{99m}Tc-DMSA is indicated in the assessment of reflux nephropathy.
   b. ^{99m}Tc-DMSA images are acquired 40 minutes after injection.
   c. upper pole scarring is better seen on posterior DMSA images.
   d. direct radionuclide micturating cystography utilises ^{99m}Tc-MAG 3.
   e. direct radionuclide micturating cystography is as sensitive as conventional MCUG for detecting reflux.

4. **Extralobar bronchopulmonary sequestration:**
   a. is associated with congenital diaphragmatic hernia.
   b. is more often right-sided.
   c. demonstrates air bronchograms on chest radiographs.
   d. takes arterial supply directly from the aorta.
   e. is associated with pectus excavatum.

5. **Cyanosis with pulmonary plethora is a feature of:**
   a. patent ductus arteriosus.
   b. truncus arteriosus.
   c. total anomalous pulmonary venous drainage.
   d. double-outlet right ventricle.
   e. tetralogy of Fallot.

6. **Regarding neonatal pneumonia:**

   a. group B *Streptococcus* infections are a common cause.
   b. pleural effusions occur frequently.
   c. *Candida* often results in an interstitial pattern on chest radiographs.
   d. pneumomediastinum is a recognised complication.
   e. *Chlamydia* often produces a bronchopneumonic pattern of consolidation.

7. **The following fractures have a high specificity for non-accidental injury:**

   a. spinous process fracture.
   b. mid-clavicular fracture.
   c. linear parietal skull fracture.
   d. rib fracture.
   e. scapular fracture.

8. **Concerning slipped capital femoral epiphysis:**

   a. there is an association with renal osteodystrophy.
   b. it is bilateral in 1–10%.
   c. the epiphysis displaces anteromedially.
   d. it is best assessed by a frog-leg lateral view.
   e. osteoarthritis is a late sequel in most cases.

9. **In children with rickets:**

   a. the epiphyses are cupped and frayed.
   b. changes are best demonstrated in the wrists and knees.
   c. a periosteal reaction is a recognised finding.
   d. narrowing of the physeal plates occurs.
   e. frontal bossing is a feature.

10. **Necrotising enterocolitis:**

    a. occurs only in premature infants.
    b. commonly involves the terminal ileum.
    c. is a contraindication to barium enema.
    d. is fatal once portal vein gas is visible at radiography.
    e. results in ascites at US.

11. In children with intussusception:

a. the ileocolic form is most common.
b. a pathological lead point is identified in most cases.
c. a pseudokidney appearance is seen in longitudinal section with US.
d. pneumatic reduction is successful in 70–90% of uncomplicated cases.
e. there is a post reduction recurrence rate of 25%.

12. Concerning congenital biliary atresia:

a. US shows intrahepatic bile duct dilatation.
b. the extrahepatic bile ducts are involved in most cases.
c. the 'triangular cord' sign at US is highly suggestive.
d. the gallbladder is small or absent.
e. no bowel activity is seen after 24 hours at ^{99m}Tc-HIDA scintigraphy.

13. The following are true of neuroblastoma:

a. calcification is seen at CT in 80–90%.
b. it commonly invades the adjacent vessels.
c. the primary tumour takes up ^{99m}Tc-MDP.
d. MIBG scintigraphy is more sensitive than MDP for cortical bone metastases.
e. an adrenal mass is the commonest site.

14. Concerning multicystic dysplastic kidney:

a. most cases are unilateral.
b. there is an association with ureteric atresia.
c. ^{99m}Tc-MAG 3 scintigraphy is usually unremarkable.
d. the cysts intercommunicate.
e. central sinus echoes are absent at US.

15. Regarding cryptorchidism:

a. the testis usually lies in the inguinal canal.
b. the risk of torsion is increased.
c. teratoma is the commonest associated tumour.
d. there is an association with testicular microlithiasis.
e. the risk of malignancy in the contralateral testis is increased.

16. **Regarding the US of neonatal brain haemorrhage:**

 a. germinal matrix haemorrhage does not occur after the seventh day of life.
 b. haemorrhage becomes less reflective with time.
 c. subependymal cysts are pathognomonic of previous haemorrhage.
 d. most babies with Papile grade II haemorrhage have long-term neurological sequelae.
 e. Papile grade III haemorrhages involve the brain parenchyma.

17. **The following are causes of widening of the cranial sutures:**

 a. cleidocranial dysplasia.
 b. achondroplasia.
 c. lead intoxication.
 d. osteogenesis imperfecta.
 e. sickle cell anaemia.

18. **The following are true of scoliosis:**

 a. most cases are idiopathic.
 b. juvenile scoliosis is usually convex to the left.
 c. scoliosis occurs in most patients with syringomyelia.
 d. headache is an indication for MRI in presumed idiopathic scoliosis.
 e. osteoid osteoma is a recognised cause.

19. **Radiological features of Down's syndrome include:**

 a. hypoplastic sinuses.
 b. premature closure of cranial sutures.
 c. atlantoaxial subluxation.
 d. aberrant right subclavian artery.
 e. duodenal atresia.

20. **The following are recognised skeletal manifestations of the mucopolysaccharidoses:**

 a. frontal bossing in Hurler's syndrome.
 b. enlarged diaphyses in Hurler's syndrome.
 c. a narrowed femoral neck in Morquio's syndrome.
 d. short metacarpals in Morquio's syndrome.
 e. flaring of the iliac wings in both Hunter's and Morquio's syndromes.

Module Five: Examination Two – Answers

1. Answers

a. **False** – it increases noise.
b. **False** – they are removed by an amplitude demodulator, or by the analogue-to-digital converter.
c. **False** – 8-bit ADCs have an output of $2^8 = 256$ numbers.
d. **True**
e. **False** – they are usually curved to enhance contrast resolution for a particular tissue, according to the application.

(Dendy & Heaton pp355–358)

2. Answers

a. **True**
b. **True**
c. **False** – the left lobe is usually larger.
d. **True** – or straight, lobulated, or convex.
e. **True**

(Butler et al. pp147–148)

3. Answers

a. **True**
b. **False** – 1–6 hours, free technetium is present in collecting system in first hour.
c. **True** – the upper poles are more posterior.
d. **False** – ^{99m}Tc-pertechnetate.
e. **True**

(Chapman & Nakielny 2001 pp164–172)

4. Answers

a. **True**
b. **False** – usually left-sided (80% of cases).
c. **False**
d. **True**
e. **True**

(Dähnert pp471–475)

5. Answers

a. **False** – not cyanotic, unless shunt reversal occurs.
b. **True**
c. **True**
d. **True**
e. **False** – pulmonary oligaemia is seen.

(Reeder pp460–461)

6. Answers

a. **True**
b. **False** – rare.
c. **False** – often causes progressive consolidation and cavitation.
d. **True**
e. **True**

(Dähnert p508)

7. Answers

a. **True**
b. **False** – outer third of clavicle.
c. **False**
d. **True**
e. **True**

(Grainger & Allison pp2113–2114)

8. Answers

a. **True**
b. **False** – 20–40% are bilateral.
c. **False** – posteromedially.
d. **False** – a cross table lateral is better for early slips.
e. **True** – in 90%.

(Dähnert p72)

9. Answers

a. **False** – the metaphyses are cupped and frayed.
b. **True**
c. **True**
d. **False** – widening.
e. **True**

(Dähnert p153)

10. Answers

a. **False** – may also occur in term babies.
b. **True**
c. **True**
d. **False** – this is not an indicator of imminent demise.
e. **True**

(Grainger & Allison pp1206–1208; Dähnert pp851–852)

11. Answers

a. **True**
b. **False** – 5%.
c. **True**
d. **True**
e. **False** – 5–10%.

(Sutton pp872–873)

12. Answers

a. **False** – no duct dilatation occurs, due to panductal sclerosis.
b. **True** – in 90%.
c. **True** – this is a focus of high reflectivity at the porta hepatis.
d. **True**
e. **True**

(Grainger & Allison pp1449–1451; Dähnert pp698–699)

13. Answers

a. **True**
b. **False** – vascular encasement is more common.
c. **True**
d. **False** – MDP is more sensitive, but the two are complementary.
e. **True**

(Grainger & Allison pp1483–1486)

14. Answers

a. **True** – 80–90% are unilateral.
b. **True**
c. **False** – MAG 3 scintigraphy shows absence of renal function.
d. **False** – no intercommunication occurs.
e. **True** – a characteristic feature.

(Dähnert pp927–928; Grainger & Allison p1751)

15. Answers

a. **True** – in 70–80%.
b. **True**
c. **False** – seminoma is the commonest associated tumour.
d. **True**
e. **True**

(Dogra VS, Gottlieb RH, Oka M et al. Sonography of the scrotum. *Radiology* 2003;227:18–36)

16. Answers

a. **False** – although 90% occur within 6 days.
b. **True** – although a rim of high reflectivity persists.
c. **False** – subependymal cysts also occur with viral infection.
d. **False** – less than 20%.
e. **False** – grade III denotes hydrocephalus, grade IV involves brain parenchyma.

(Dähnert pp305–307; Grainger & Allison p2471)

17. Answers

a. **True** – due to congenital underossification.
b. **False** – causes craniosynostosis.
c. **True**
d. **True** – due to congenital underossification.
e. **False** – causes craniosynostosis.

(Dähnert p173)

18. Answers

a. **True** – 85% are idiopathic.
b. **False** – usually convex to the right.
c. **True** – 70% of syringomyelias are associated with scoliosis.
d. **True**
e. **True** – causes a painful scoliosis.

(Cassar-Pullicino VN, Eisenstein SM. Imaging in scoliosis: what, why and how? *Clin Radiol* 2002;57:543–562)

19. Answers

a. **True**
b. **False** – delayed closure.
c. **True**
d. **True**
e. **True**

(Dähnert p68)

20. Answers

a. **True**
b. **True**
c. **False** – the femoral necks are widened, the femoral epiphyses are poorly formed.
d. **True**
e. **True**

(Dähnert pp119–121)

Module Five: Examination Three – Questions

1. **Concerning the components of a modern gamma camera:**

   a. diverging collimators produce a minified image.
   b. photomultiplier tubes operate at a potential difference of 120 kV.
   c. photomultiplier tubes contain argon at low pressure.
   d. pulse arithmetic circuits accept pulses within a certain energy window.
   e. image display is usually at a matrix of 512×512.

2. **The following are true of paediatric neuroanatomy as demonstrated by US:**

   a. a central reflective line in the spinal cord is due to the central canal.
   b. the conus medullaris can normally lie at the level of L3/4 in a neonate.
   c. choroid plexus may normally be seen in the third ventricle.
   d. a cavum septum vergae lies anterior to the cavum septum pellucidum.
   e. the lateral ventricles appear relatively smaller in premature than in term infants.

3. **The following radiographs are routinely performed as part of the skeletal survey for non-accidental injury:**

   a. lateral thoracolumbar spine.
   b. AP and lateral views of both upper limbs.
   c. lateral view of the cervical spine.
   d. collimated lateral views of both knees.
   e. Towne's view of the skull.

4. **Neonatal respiratory distress syndrome:**

   a. is more severe in males.
   b. is effectively excluded if the chest radiograph is normal at 12 hours.
   c. causes reticulogranular shadowing.
   d. characteristically produces symmetrical radiographic changes.
   e. which improves asymmetrically following surfactant has a poorer prognosis.

5. **Congenital lobar emphysema:**

 a. initially causes an opaque lobe.
 b. is associated with congenital heart disease.
 c. causes atelectasis of the adjacent lobes.
 d. most often occurs in the upper lobes.
 e. rarely causes respiratory distress.

6. **The following congenital anomalies indent the posterior oesophagus:**

 a. double aortic arch.
 b. aberrant left pulmonary artery.
 c. right aortic arch with aberrant left subclavian artery.
 d. left aortic arch with aberrant right subclavian artery.
 e. right aortic arch with mirror image branching.

7. **Concerning non-accidental injury:**

 a. diaphyseal fractures are more common than are metaphyseal.
 b. rib fractures are usually anterior.
 c. depressed occipital fractures are considered a specific finding.
 d. metaphyseal fractures are most common around the elbow.
 e. lamellar periosteal reaction can be a normal finding in the tibia.

8. **The following are features of juvenile chronic arthritis:**

 a. delayed closure of the epiphyseal growth plates.
 b. metacarpal periosteal new bone formation.
 c. flaring of the ribs.
 d. pleural effusions and pulmonary nodules.
 e. involvement of the small joints of the hand before large joints.

9. **Langerhans' cell histiocytosis of bone:**

 a. usually presents with lesions in multiple bones.
 b. typically involves the posterior elements of vertebrae.
 c. is usually diaphyseal in long bones.
 d. has an associated soft tissue mass at MRI in 20–30%.
 e. appears as a well-defined lesion in the early stages.

10. **CT features of hypoperfusion complex following abdominal trauma in children include:**

 a. periportal low attenuation.
 b. bowel dilatation.
 c. poor adrenal enhancement.
 d. reduced aortic calibre.
 e. intense renal enhancement.

11. Concerning meconium ileus:

a. it is the presenting feature of cystic fibrosis in 60–80%.
b. it is associated with small bowel atresia.
c. contrast enema demonstrates a dilated colon.
d. for therapeutic enema, Gastrografin should not be diluted.
e. small bowel fluid levels are a prominent radiographic finding.

12. Concerning malrotation:

a. the small bowel mesentery is longer than normal.
b. there is an association with Hirschsprung's disease.
c. finding the superior mesenteric artery to the right of the vein at US is pathognomonic.
d. the duodenojejunal junction can be displaced by colonic distension.
e. a 'corkscrew' pattern of small bowel at contrast study is a non-specific finding.

13. Annular pancreas:

a. is associated with Down's syndrome.
b. is the commonest congenital pancreatic abnormality.
c. is a recognised cause of the 'double bubble' sign.
d. is associated with an increased risk of pancreatitis.
e. is well demonstrated at CT.

14. Wilms' tumour:

a. is bilateral in 30%.
b. arises peripherally and spares the collecting system.
c. usually presents with abdominal pain.
d. frequently calcifies.
e. metastasises to lung.

15. Ureterocoeles:

a. are associated with ureteral duplication in most cases.
b. appear as a cystic extravesical mass at US.
c. can cause bladder outlet obstruction.
d. have a 'cobra head' appearance at IVU.
e. may be seen to collapse at dynamic US.

16. **At US in a 4-year-old boy, both kidneys measure 10 cm. The differential diagnosis includes:**

   a. leukaemia.
   b. Alport syndrome.
   c. Henoch–Schönlein purpura.
   d. nephroblastomatosis.
   e. bilateral duplex kidneys.

17. **Craniosynostosis:**

   a. usually involves a single suture.
   b. of the sagittal suture causes brachycephaly.
   c. occurs in hyperparathyroidism.
   d. is associated with raised intracranial pressure.
   e. of the metopic suture results in trigonocephaly.

18. **The following occur in Sturge–Weber syndrome:**

   a. cortical atrophy.
   b. enlargement of the choroid plexus.
   c. cortical arteriovenous malformations.
   d. subdural fluid collections.
   e. cranial asymmetry.

19. **Concerning the intracranial features of non-accidental injury (NAI):**

   a. skull fractures can be dated by the extent of callus formation.
   b. subdural haematomas are often interhemispheric.
   c. cysts are seen at transcranial US following shear injury.
   d. the basal ganglia are of lower attenuation than surrounding brain following hypoxic damage.
   e. subdural haematoma without skull fracture is suspicious for NAI.

20. **The following are features of congenital rubella infection:**

   a. irregular metaphyseal margins.
   b. porencephalic cysts.
   c. periostitis.
   d. pneumonitis.
   e. hepatosplenomegaly.

Module Five: Examination Three – Answers

1. Answers

a. **True**
b. **False** – 1200 V, most often.
c. **False** – they are evacuated.
d. **False** – they calculate the X, Y and Z components of each pulse, the pulse height analyser then 'chooses' which pulses to accept or reject.
e. **False** – the common matrices are 64 × 64, 128 × 128 and 256 × 256.

(Dendy & Heaton pp168–171)

2. Answers

a. **False** – it is due to the interface of anterior commissure and anterior fissure.
b. **False** – the cord does not normally lie below the superior endplate of L3.
c. **True**
d. **False** – posterior.
e. **False** – appear relatively larger.

(Butler et al. pp417–418)

3. Answers

a. **True**
b. **False** – AP views only, also of both lower limbs.
c. **False**
d. **True** – also of both ankles.
e. **False** – frontal and lateral views are routine, Towne's view only if occipital injury.

(Rao P, Carty H. Non-accidental injury: review of the radiology. *Clin Radiol* 1999;54:11–24)

4. Answers

a. **True** – also more common in boys.
b. **True** – the chest radiograph is usually abnormal by 6 hours.
c. **True** – also air bronchograms.
d. **False** – asymmetric changes are well recognised.
e. **False** – this is a good prognostic sign.

(Grainger & Allison pp634–635; Sutton pp256–257)

5. Answers

a. **True** – due to retained fluid.
b. **True** – particularly with VSD and PDA.
c. **True**
d. **True**
e. **False** – occurs in 90% of affected babies within 6 months.

(Dähnert p478)

6. Answers

a. **True** – large posterior indentation.
b. **False** – anterior oesophageal indentation.
c. **True** – small indentation.
d. **True** – small indentation.
e. **False** – no vascular ring is present, so no oesophageal indentation occurs.

(Dähnert pp579–580)

7. Answers

a. **True** – by a factor of four.
b. **False** – usually posterior.
c. **True**
d. **False** – metaphyseal fractures are most common around the knees and ankles.
e. **True** – between six weeks and six months.

(Grainger & Allison pp2115–2118)

8. Answers

a. **False** – early closure.
b. **True** – also phalangeal periosteal new bone.
c. **False** – narrow, 'ribbon' ribs occur.
d. **True**
e. **False** – large joints are involved before small joints.

(Grainger & Allison pp2144–2145; Dähnert pp152–153)

9. Answers

a. **False** – monostotic in 75%.
b. **False** – almost always in the vertebral body.
c. **True** – in 60%.
d. **True** – high signal at T2-weighting.
e. **False** – initially poorly-defined and aggressive-looking, becomes more well-defined with time.

(Kilborn TN, Teh J, Goodman TR. Paediatric manifestations of Langerhans cell histiocytosis: a review of the clinical and radiological findings. *Clin Radiol* 2003;58:269–278)

10. Answers

a. **True**
b. **True** – and bowel wall thickening.
c. **False** – marked adrenal enhancement.
d. **True** – also IVC.
e. **True**

(Grainger & Allison p1219)

11. Answers

a. **False** – presenting feature in 10–15%.
b. **True**
c. **False** – a microcolon is found at enema.
d. **False** – half-strength Gastrografin is effective and safer.
e. **False** – they are frequently absent.

(Grainger & Allison pp1210–1212)

12. Answers

a. **False** – shorter than normal, increasing the risk of volvulus.
b. **True**
c. **False** – this pattern may occur in otherwise normal individuals.
d. **True**
e. **False** – it is pathognomonic of malrotation.

(Grainger & Allison pp1203–1205; Dähnert pp843–844)

13. Answers

a. **True** – also duodenal and oesophageal atresia, and imperforate anus.
b. **False** – pancreas divisum is the commonest congenital abnormality.
c. **True** – due to duodenal obstruction.
d. **True**
e. **True** – pancreatic tissue is seen to surround the second part of the duodenum.

(Grainger & Allison pp1345–1346; Dähnert pp681–682)

14. Answers

a. **False** – 12%.
b. **True**
c. **False** – bulging flank is the commonest sign.
d. **False** – does in 5–15%.
e. **True**

(Dähnert pp984–985)

15. Answers

a. **True** – ureteral duplication is present in up to 75%.
b. **False** – intravesical cystic mass.
c. **True** – by prolapsing into the urethra.
d. **True** – the classical appearance.
e. **True** – due to ureteric peristalsis.

(Berrocal T, Lopez-Pereira P, Arjonilla A et al. Anomalies of the distal ureter, bladder and urethra in children: embryologic, radiologic and pathologic features. *Radiographics* 2002;22:1139–1164)

16. Answers

a. **True** – a recognised cause of bilateral renal enlargement.
b. **False** – the kidneys are small in this disorder (hereditary chronic nephritis).
c. **True**
d. **True**
e. **True**

(Dähnert p873)

17. Answers

a. **True**
b. **False** – this causes scaphocephaly.
c. **True**
d. **True** – a recognised complication of craniosynostosis.
e. **True**

(Aviv RI, Rodger E, Hall CM. Craniosynostosis. *Clin Radiol* 2002;57:93–102)

18. Answers

a. **True**
b. **True** – also calcification of choroid plexus.
c. **False** – leptomeningeal AVMs occur.
d. **True**
e. **True** – due to hemiatrophy.

(Herron J, Darrah R, Quaghebeur G. Intracranial manifestations of the neurocutaneous syndromes. *Clin Radiol* 2000;55:82–98)

19. Answers

a. **False** – skull fractures do not heal by callus formation.
b. **True**
c. **True**
d. **False** – they are of higher attenuation, the 'acute reversal sign'.
e. **True**

(Rao P, Carty H. Non-accidental injury: a review of the radiology. *Clin Radiol* 1999;54:11–24)

20. Answers

a. **True**
b. **True**
c. **False**
d. **True**
e. **True**

(Dähnert p155)

MODULE SIX

Neuroradiology and Head and Neck

Time Allowed: 1.5 hours

Module Six: Examination One – Questions

1. **In positron emission tomography:**

   a. a pair of positrons collide, emitting two 511 keV gamma photons.
   b. coincidence detection is necessary.
   c. increased collimation is required at the detectors.
   d. resolution deteriorates with increasing patient depth.
   e. bismuth germanate detectors are used.

2. **The following statements are true:**

   a. the anterior spinal artery is formed by branches of the vertebral arteries.
   b. the lumbosacral intervertebral disc is the largest in height.
   c. the thoracic superior articular facets face posterolaterally.
   d. the foramen transversarium of C7 does not transmit the vertebral artery.
   e. the ligamentum flavum becomes thicker caudally in the spine.

3. **The following are true:**

   a. the foramen ovale transmits the maxillary branch of the trigeminal nerve.
   b. the foramen of Luschka opens into the cerebellopontine angle.
   c. the trochlear nerve emerges from the dorsum of the pons.
   d. the claustrum lies between the insula and extreme capsule.
   e. the basal vein of Rosenthal is an unpaired midline vein.

4. **The following are true regarding myelography:**

   a. lumbar myelography should be avoided within 7 days of lumbar puncture.
   b. diatrizoate meglumine is a suitable contrast agent.
   c. the maximum dose of contrast is 6 g iodine.
   d. a smaller spinal needle does not reduce the incidence of headache.
   e. contrast remains loculated at the needle tip after inadvertent extradural injection.

5. **Cerebral metastases:**

   a. are most common in the deep white matter.
   b. from melanoma return high signal at T1-weighted MRI.
   c. from breast are commonly hyperdense.
   d. are the commonest supratentorial mass lesions.
   e. typically enhance following IV contrast.

6. **Primary cerebral lymphoma in immunocompetent patients:**

   a. is of high attenuation at unenhanced CT.
   b. shows marked ring enhancement.
   c. often contains central necrosis at MRI.
   d. shows increased uptake at ^{201}Tl SPECT.
   e. often abuts the ependymal surface.

7. **Intracranial tuberculosis:**

   a. causes dural thickening.
   b. in the UK is more common in children than in adults.
   c. frequently involves the brainstem.
   d. shows strong contrast enhancement.
   e. when calcified, is often visible at skull radiography.

8. **Regarding MRI findings in multiple sclerosis:**

   a. cortical lesions are more conspicuous than white matter lesions.
   b. plaques can show ring enhancement.
   c. the corpus callosum is characteristically spared.
   d. plaques are usually perpendicular to the long axis of the spinal cord.
   e. leptomeningeal enhancement is a common finding.

9. **Regarding intracranial arteriovenous malformations:**

   a. the majority are infratentorial.
   b. mass effect is a common finding.
   c. lesions are of mixed attenuation at CT.
   d. the affected arteries are thick-walled.
   e. the risk of haemorrhage is 2–5% per annum.

10. **In the investigation of patients with subarachnoid haemorrhage (SAH):**

    a. the sensitivity of CT at seven days is only 50%.
    b. all patients have xanthochromic CSF after 12 hours.
    c. CT is more sensitive than MRI in the acute stage.
    d. FLAIR MRI is superior to CT for subacute SAH.
    e. four-vessel cerebral angiography is negative in 40–60%.

11. **Causes of cerebellar atrophy include:**

    a. paraneoplastic syndrome.
    b. phenytoin.
    c. alcohol misuse.
    d. Friedreich's ataxia.
    e. hereditary haemorrhagic telangiectasia.

12. Regarding hydrocephalus:

a. CSF flow is obstructed in communicating hydrocephalus.
b. all ventricles are dilated in communicating hydrocephalus.
c. Dandy–Walker syndrome causes non-communicating hydrocephalus.
d. infection most often causes non-communicating hydrocephalus.
e. choroid plexus papilloma is a recognised cause.

13. The 'empty sella':

a. results in a small pituitary fossa on a lateral skull radiograph.
b. usually contains CSF.
c. is associated with papilloedema.
d. is asymptomatic in the majority.
e. can follow involution of a pituitary tumour.

14. Ependymomas:

a. are most common in the third ventricle.
b. cause hydrocephalus.
c. contain cystic areas at enhanced CT.
d. rarely show calcification.
e. invade the brain parenchyma through the ventricular walls.

15. Cranial nerve schwannomas:

a. are more common on sensory than motor nerves.
b. infiltrate the nerve.
c. enhance poorly following IV contrast.
d. are the commonest lesion of the cerebellopontine angle.
e. contain cystic areas at T2-weighted MRI.

16. A lateral radiograph of the thoracic spine shows multiple collapsed vertebrae. Possible causes include:

a. syphilis.
b. sickle cell disease.
c. renal osteodystrophy.
d. osteomalacia.
e. osteopoikilosis.

17. The following are true of percutaneous vertebroplasty:

a. myelomatous compression fractures are an indication.
b. fractures involving the posterior vertebral elements are a contraindication.
c. a transient fever is to be expected.
d. pain relief should not be expected for at least seven days.
e. pulmonary embolus is a recognised complication.

18. **Six weeks after lumbar discectomy, the following MRI findings are normal:**

  a. enhancement of the intervertebral disc space.
  b. nerve root enhancement.
  c. epidural soft tissue with mass effect.
  d. facet joint enhancement.
  e. cauda equina adhesions.

19. **Recognised causes of calcification of intervertebral discs include:**

  a. alkaptonuria.
  b. Klippel–Feil syndrome.
  c. diffuse idiopathic skeletal hyperostosis.
  d. haemochromatosis.
  e. Wilson's disease.

20. **In patients with diastematomyelia:**

  a. the cervical and upper thoracic spine is the commonest site.
  b. a bony spur can divide the spinal canal.
  c. there is an association with myelomeningocoele.
  d. the conus is frequently low-lying.
  e. the hemicords can have separate dural sheaths.

21. **The following are causes of loss of the lamina dura of teeth:**

  a. hyperparathyroidism.
  b. Cushing's syndrome.
  c. Paget's disease.
  d. scleroderma.
  e. osteoporosis.

22. **The rectus muscles of the eye are enlarged by:**

  a. acromegaly.
  b. tuberculosis.
  c. Sjögren's syndrome.
  d. orbital cellulitis.
  e. cavernous sinus thrombosis.

23. **Following IV contrast, perineural enhancement of the optic nerve is seen in the following:**

  a. carcinomatous infiltration.
  b. multiple sclerosis.
  c. optic meningioma.
  d. lymphoma.
  e. orbital pseudotumour.

24. The following are features of orbital pseudotumour:

a. bilateral involvement in most cases.
b. lacrimal gland swelling.
c. scleral enhancement at CT following IV contrast.
d. rapid response to corticosteroids.
e. diffuse swelling of extra-ocular muscles at MRI.

25. The following are true of head and neck anatomy:

a. the superior orbital fissure opens into the middle cranial fossa.
b. the scutum forms the medial wall of the epitympanum.
c. the superior and inferior compartments of the temporomandibular joint do not communicate.
d. the frontal sinus drains via the hiatus semilunaris.
e. the articulation between cricoid and arytenoid cartilages is synovial.

26. Causes of temporal bone sclerosis include:

a. Paget's disease.
b. fibrous dysplasia.
c. meningioma.
d. osteogenesis imperfecta.
e. metastases.

27. Regarding sinus imaging prior to endoscopic sinus surgery:

a. it is mandatory.
b. CT scans are obtained in the coronal plane.
c. bone sclerosis indicates acute sinusitis.
d. secretions in acute sinusitis have attenuations of 10–25 HU.
e. in chronic sinusitis, secretions have higher attenuation than in acute disease.

28. The following are true of thyroid scintigraphy:

a. Graves' disease shows diffuse uptake of ^{123}I.
b. toxic nodules manifest as an area of intense activity.
c. in ^{131}I therapy, a solitary nodule needs a greater dose than Graves' disease.
d. demonstration of a 'cold' nodule within a toxic gland is indication for FNAC.
e. a pyramidal lobe is more easily seen with thyrotoxicosis than in the euthyroid state.

29. **The following US features suggest that an enlarged lymph node is benign:**

a. high reflectivity at the hilum.
b. rounded shape.
c. distal acoustic enhancement.
d. a central vascular pattern at power Doppler.
e. punctate calcification.

30. **Metastases to the thyroid:**

a. most often arise from the lung.
b. are well-defined at US.
c. are frequently calcified.
d. are of low reflectivity at US.
e. are usually solitary.

Module Six: Examination One – Answers

1. Answers

- **a. False** – a positron collides with an electron to produce the annihilation radiation.
- **b. True**
- **c. False** – little or no collimation is needed as coincidence detection eliminates stray or scattered radiation.
- **d. False** – it remains the same.
- **e. True**

(Dendy & Heaton pp274–275; Farr & Allisy-Roberts pp144–146)

2. Answers

- **a. True**
- **b. False** – the L5/S1 disc is slightly smaller than the L4/5 disc.
- **c. True**
- **d. True** – transmits the vertebral vein.
- **e. True**

(Butler et al. pp306–328)

3. Answers

- **a. False** – transmits the mandibular branch, and the accessory meningeal artery.
- **b. True**
- **c. False** – dorsum of the midbrain.
- **d. False** – between the putamen and insula.
- **e. False** – it is a bilateral structure.

(Butler et al. pp22–58)

4. Answers

- **a. True** – due to subdural accumulation of CSF.
- **b. False** – it is ionic; only iopamidol, iohexol and iotrolan are licensed.
- **c. False** – 3 g iodine (i.e. 10 ml of 300 mg ml^{-1}).
- **d. False**
- **e. False** – this occurs with subdural injection.

(Chapman & Nakielny 2001 pp312–320)

5. Answers

- **a. False** – usually occur at the grey–white matter junction.
- **b. True**
- **c. False** – usually of similar density to brain.
- **d. False** – glioma is more common than metastases.
- **e. True** – enhancement is an almost universal feature.

(Grainger & Allison p2333; Haaga et al. pp195–198)

6. Answers

a. **True** – the classical appearance.
b. **False** – enhancement is usually uniform, ring enhancement is seen in immunocompromised patients.
c. **False** – uncommon in immunocompetent patients.
d. **True** – can be used to differentiate from toxoplasmosis.
e. **True** – a common late finding.

(Grainger & Allison pp2332–2333; Haaga et al. pp177–178; Dähnert p298)

7. Answers

a. **True**
b. **False** – more common in adults in developed countries.
c. **False** – brainstem disease is infrequent (2–8%).
d. **True**
e. **False** – not usually seen, but can be detected with CT.

(Sutton p1785; Grainger & Allison pp2379–2380)

8. Answers

a. **False** – white matter lesions are more conspicuous.
b. **True**
c. **False** – it is commonly involved.
d. **False** – usually parallel.
e. **False** – leptomeningeal enhancement suggests an alternative diagnosis.

(Pretorius PM, Quaghebeur G. The role of MRI in the diagnosis of MS. *Clin Radiol* 2003;58:434–448)

9. Answers

a. **False** – 90% are supratentorial.
b. **False** – rarely cause mass effect.
c. **True** – in 60%.
d. **False** – thin-walled.
e. **True**

(Dähnert p263)

10. Answers

a. **True** – it is 98% sensitive on day one.
b. **True** – xanthochromia persists for two weeks.
c. **True**
d. **True**
e. **False** – only 15–20% are negative.

(Hoggard N, Wilkinson ID, Paley MNI et al. Imaging of haemorrhagic stroke. *Clin Radiol* 2002;57:957–968)

11. Answers

a. **True**
b. **True**
c. **True**
d. **True**
e. **False** – ataxia telangiectasia causes cerebellar atrophy, however.

(Sutton p1797)

12. Answers

a. **True**
b. **True**
c. **True**
d. **False** – communicating.
e. **True**

(Sutton p1728)

13. Answers

a. **False** – larger than normal.
b. **True**
c. **True** – secondary to benign intracranial hypertension.
d. **True**
e. **True**

(Grainger & Allison p2345)

14. Answers

a. **False** – 65% occur in fourth ventricle.
b. **True**
c. **True** – in up to half of fourth ventricle tumours, and in over 80% of supratentorial.
d. **False** – up to half show calcification.
e. **False** – spread via the ventricular system.

(Haaga et al. pp147–150)

15. Answers

a. **True**
b. **False** – they arise eccentrically.
c. **False** – avid enhancement occurs.
d. **True**
e. **True** – when large.

(Grainger & Allison p2339; Haaga et al. pp162–165)

16. Answers

a. **True** – secondary to osteomyelitis or neuropathy.
b. **True**
c. **True** – due to hyperparathyroidism.
d. **True**
e. **False**

(Reeder p201)

17. Answers

a. **True** – also osteoporotic and metastatic fractures.
b. **True** – also bleeding diathesis, lack of definite level of collapse and inability to lie prone.
c. **True** – due to polymerisation of polymethyl methacrylate (PMM).
d. **False** – pain relief usually occurs with 24 hours.
e. **True** – due to venous leakage of PMM.

(Peh WCG, Gilula LA. Percutaneous vertebroplasty: indications, contraindications and technique. *Br J Radiol* 2003;76:69–75)

18. Answers

a. **True** – in 67% for up to six weeks.
b. **True** – in 20–62% for three to six weeks.
c. **True** – due to oedema or haematoma.
d. **True** – a local response to dissection.
e. **True** – quite common, but resolve with time.

(Babar S, Saifuddin A. MRI of the post-discectomy lumbar spine. *Clin Radiol* 2002;57:969–981)

19. Answers

a. **True**
b. **True** – and other causes of block vertebra.
c. **True**
d. **True**
e. **True**

(Reeder pp219–220)

20. Answers

a. **False** – lower thoracic and upper lumbar, usually.
b. **True** – in fewer than 50%.
c. **True**
d. **True** – below L2 in 75%.
e. **True** – in 40%.

(Dähnert p202)

21. Answers

a. **True**
b. **True**
c. **True**
d. **True**
e. **True**

(Chapman & Nakielny 2003 p391)

22. Answers

a. **True**
b. **True**
c. **True**
d. **True**
e. **True** – secondary to increased venous pressure.

(Reeder pp111–112)

23. Answers

a. **True**
b. **True**
c. **True**
d. **True**
e. **True**

(Reeder p111)

24. Answers

a. **False** – over half of cases are unilateral.
b. **True**
c. **True**
d. **True**
e. **True** – cf. thyroid eye disease.

(Grainger & Allison p2530)

25. Answers

a. **True**
b. **False** – lateral wall.
c. **True** – divided by a fibrocartilaginous disc.
d. **True**
e. **True**

(Butler et al. pp86–112)

26. Answers

a. **True**
b. **True**
c. **True**
d. **True**
e. **True**

(Dähnert p350)

27. Answers

a. **True** – there is a medico-legal requirement for imaging.
b. **True**
c. **False** – chronic disease.
d. **True**
e. **True** – 60–80 HU, typically.

(Sutton p1521)

28. Answers

- a. **True**
- b. **True**
- c. **True**
- d. **True**
- e. **True**

(Sutton p1505)

29. Answers

- a. **True**
- b. **False** – elliptical shape.
- c. **False** – 90% of lymphomas show this.
- d. **True**
- e. **False** – this suggests metastases from medullary thyroid carcinoma.

(Ahuja & Evans pp75–81)

30. Answers

- a. **False** – melanoma most common (39%), breast next (21%).
- b. **True**
- c. **False** – non-calcified.
- d. **True**
- e. **True**

(Ahuja & Evans pp51–52)

Module Six: Examination Two – Questions

1. **Single photon emission computed tomography (SPECT):**

   a. results in superior spatial resolution to conventional scintigraphy.
   b. can be performed with an elliptical orbit.
   c. typically acquires data at 15 degree intervals around the patient.
   d. can only be performed with dual-headed gamma cameras.
   e. is performed with the collimator removed from the gamma camera.

2. **The following are normal causes of intracranial calcification:**

   a. choroid plexus.
   b. dura mater.
   c. Pacchionian bodies.
   d. the lens.
   e. habenular commissure.

3. **The following structures border the third ventricle:**

   a. thalamus.
   b. hypothalamus.
   c. caudate nucleus.
   d. pineal.
   e. habenular commissure.

4. **With respect to skull radiography:**

   a. the side of interest should be closest to the film.
   b. the centring point of a lateral view is over the pituitary fossa.
   c. the PA view is taken with the central ray tilted 20 degrees cranially.
   d. the Towne's view is taken with the central ray tilted 30 degrees caudally.
   e. the PA view is taken with the orbitomeatal line horizontal.

5. **The following primary tumours give rise to haemorrhagic brain metastases:**

   a. colon.
   b. melanoma.
   c. thyroid.
   d. lung.
   e. choriocarcinoma.

6. **Colloid cysts:**

   a. arise from the septum pellucidum.
   b. are thick-walled lesions.
   c. are of higher attenuation than CSF at CT.
   d. show calcification in 20–30% of cases.
   e. can be hypointense at T2-weighted MRI.

7. **The following are features of herpes simplex encephalitis:**

   a. unilateral temporal lobe swelling.
   b. patchy gyral enhancement.
   c. localised cerebral atrophy.
   d. significant mass effect.
   e. haemorrhagic lesions.

8. **HIV-related progressive multifocal leukoencephalopathy:**

   a. occurs due to treatment with reverse transcriptase inhibitors.
   b. presents with limb weakness.
   c. causes subcortical T2-bright lesions.
   d. involves the basal ganglia.
   e. causes enhancing lesions.

9. **The following are true of cerebral venous sinus thrombosis:**

   a. symptoms usually evolve gradually over days.
   b. headache is the commonest presenting feature.
   c. no predisposing factor is found in most cases.
   d. the thrombosed sinus is hyperdense at unenhanced CT.
   e. venous infarction shows enhancement with IV Gd-DTPA.

10. **Regarding subdural haematomas (SDH):**

    a. they are often bilateral in infants.
    b. extension across the midline occurs.
    c. the inner margin is usually convex.
    d. epilepsy predisposes to chronic SDH.
    e. subacute subdural haematomas are best seen at MRI.

11. **The following are causes of basal ganglia calcification:**

    a. hyperparathyroidism.
    b. neurofibromatosis.
    c. toxoplasmosis.
    d. carbon monoxide poisoning.
    e. Wilson's disease.

12. Glioblastoma multiforme:

a. is commonly multifocal.
b. spreads via the CSF more often than via the corpus callosum.
c. appears heterogeneous at unenhanced CT.
d. is associated with significant oedema.
e. is well-defined at T2-weighted MRI.

13. Regarding spinal metastases:

a. medulloblastoma is commonest source of 'drop' metastases.
b. most occur to the cervical region.
c. cord metastases tend to be ventral in distribution.
d. CT myelography is more sensitive than contrast enhanced MRI.
e. involved nerve roots are thickened and nodular.

14. The following are true of cerebral pyogenic abscesses:

a. contrast enhancement is suppressed by corticosteroids.
b. most occur in the temporal lobe.
c. frontal abscesses are associated with dural tears.
d. cyanotic heart disease is a predisposing factor.
e. contrast-enhanced CT is more sensitive than MRI.

15. Ring enhancing lesions at MRI are a feature of:

a. glioblastoma multiforme.
b. fungal abscess.
c. resolving cerebral infarction.
d. craniopharyngioma.
e. cysticercosis.

16. Regarding epidural haematomas of the spine:

a. most cases are secondary to an underlying vertebral fracture.
b. the cervical spine is the commonest site.
c. they are best seen on axial images.
d. they are usually located in the posterior epidural space.
e. osteomyelitis or discitis is usually present.

17. Atlanto-axial instability is a recognised complication of:

a. rheumatoid arthritis.
b. juvenile chronic arthritis.
c. retropharyngeal cellulitis.
d. tuberculosis.
e. Down's syndrome.

18. **When imaging the lumbar spine with MRI:**

a. disc bulges increase in the erect-extended position.
b. dural sac cross-sectional area is increased by axial compression.
c. supine extension-rotation reduces the thickness of the ligamentum flavum.
d. the sagittal diameter of the central canal increases in the erect-flexed position.
e. axial loading accentuates lateral recess stenosis.

19. **Increased vertebral ('corduroy') trabeculation of vertebral bodies is a recognised feature of:**

a. haemangioma.
b. osteoporosis.
c. anaemia.
d. fluorosis.
e. melorheostosis.

20. **Regarding pyogenic discitis:**

a. multiple level involvement is common.
b. disc space narrowing is the earliest radiographic sign.
c. enhancement occurs in the disc space but not the vertebral body.
d. bone scintigraphy is more sensitive than MRI.
e. it is most common in the lumbar spine.

21. **The following are causes of 'floating' teeth on plain radiographs:**

a. Langerhans' cell histiocytosis.
b. hypoparathyroidism.
c. Paget's disease.
d. multiple myeloma.
e. metastases.

22. **The orbit is enlarged in the following conditions:**

a. thyrotoxicosis.
b. neurofibromatosis.
c. Paget's disease.
d. frontal sinus mucocoele.
e. optic nerve glioma.

23. **Carotid–cavernous fistulas:**

a. are most often post-traumatic in origin.
b. are associated with oculomotor nerve palsy.
c. cause enlargement of the superior ophthalmic vein at CT.
d. drain via cortical veins in 30–40%.
e. can be treated by microcatheter injection of thrombin.

24. Calcification in the orbit occurs with:

a. orbital varices.
b. glaucoma.
c. radiation therapy.
d. previous trauma.
e. hypothyroidism.

25. When imaging the thyroid with scintigraphy:

a. ^{99m}Tc-pertechnetate is trapped and organified.
b. a drink of water is necessary before imaging with ^{123}I.
c. a pinhole collimator is suitable.
d. imaging is performed 2 hours after injection of ^{99m}Tc-pertechnetate.
e. ^{123}I can be administered orally.

26. Cholesteatoma:

a. is most often of the primary form.
b. is a cause of facial nerve palsy.
c. enhances with IV Gd-DTPA.
d. causes ossicular destruction.
e. causes sagittal sinus thrombosis.

27. Sinus mucocoeles:

a. are most common in the ethmoids.
b. expand the sinus cavity.
c. have a surrounding zone of sclerosis.
d. show homogenous enhancement at MRI.
e. can contain signal void at T2-weighted MRI.

28. The following are true of medullary thyroid carcinoma:

a. it is associated with multiple endocrine neoplasia.
b. a high reflectivity nodule at US is typical.
c. nodal metastases are seen in 50% on presentation.
d. it tends to affect the lower third of the thyroid.
e. involved nodes are of low reflectivity with echogenic foci.

29. Juvenile angiofibroma:

a. is the commonest benign tumour of the nasopharynx.
b. requires biopsy for diagnosis.
c. widens the pterygomaxillary fissure.
d. shows delayed enhancement at CT.
e. enhances markedly with IV Gd-DTPA.

30. **Regarding imaging of the parathyroids:**

a. parathyroid adenomas are of low reflectivity at US.
b. calcification is common within parathyroid adenomas.
c. parathyroid cysts usually occur below the inferior thyroid border.
d. parathyroid cysts are thick-walled.
e. most parathyroid lesions are hypervascular.

Module Six: Examination Two – Answers

1. Answers

a. **False** – spatial resolution is inferior to conventional scintigraphy.
b. **True** – to reduce the camera–patient gap, and so improve resolution.
c. **False** – data are acquired every 3–6 degrees.
d. **False** – single-headed camera SPECT is possible.
e. **False**

(Dendy & Heaton pp272–273; Farr & Allisy-Roberts pp143–144)

2. Answers

a. **True**
b. **True**
c. **True**
d. **True**
e. **True**

(Sutton pp1621–1622)

3. Answers

a. **True**
b. **True**
c. **False** – borders lateral ventricle.
d. **True**
e. **True**

(Butler et al. pp39–41)

4. Answers

a. **True**
b. **True**
c. **False** – 20 degrees caudally.
d. **True**
e. **False** – vertically.

(Sutton pp1617–1621)

5. Answers

a. **False**
b. **True**
c. **True**
d. **True**
e. **True** – also breast.

(Reeder p46)

6. Answers

- a. **True** – arise from the inferior portion and protrude into the anterior portion of the third ventricle.
- b. **False** – thin-walled.
- c. **True**
- d. **False** – rarely calcify.
- e. **True** – due to the paramagnetic effects of magnesium, copper and iron.

(Dähnert p271)

7. Answers

- a. **True** – initially unilateral, becoming bilateral later.
- b. **True**
- c. **True**
- d. **True**
- e. **True**

(Chapman & Nakielny 2003 pp412–413; Sutton p1792)

8. Answers

- a. **False** – occurs due to reactivation of the JC or SV40 viruses.
- b. **True** – the commonest presentation.
- c. **True** – which extend into the gyral cores.
- d. **True** – due to presence of traversing white matter tracts.
- e. **False**

(Grainger & Allison pp2386–2387)

9. Answers

- a. **True**
- b. **True**
- c. **False** – predisposing factors are found in 80%: pregnancy, the oral contraceptive pill and the puerperium are the most common.
- d. **True** – in 20–55%.
- e. **True**

(Connor SEJ, Jarosz JM. Magnetic resonance imaging of cerebral venous sinus thrombosis. *Clin Radiol* 2002;57:449–461)

10. Answers

- a. **True** – 80–85% of cases.
- b. **False**
- c. **False** – concave.
- d. **True**
- e. **True** – T1 MRI has high sensitivity for methaemoglobin.

(Dähnert pp321–323)

11. Answers

a. **True** – also hypoparathyroidism, pseudohypoparathyroidism and pseudopseudohypoparathyroidism.
b. **True**
c. **True**
d. **True**
e. **False** – causes low attenuation lesions in the basal ganglia.

(Dähnert p197; Reeder p40)

12. Answers

a. **False** – multifocal in 2–5%.
b. **False** – callosal spread occurs in 36% versus < 2% for CSF spread.
c. **True** – due to necrosis.
d. **True**
e. **False** – poorly-defined, no imaging modality can demonstrate the full extent of the lesion.

(Sutton p1743; Dähnert p282)

13. Answers

a. **True** – 33% of all cases.
b. **False** – 75% occur in the lumbosacral area.
c. **False** – dorsal spinal cord, reflecting direction of flow of CSF.
d. **False** – contrast-enhanced MR is more sensitive.
e. **True**

(Dähnert p214)

14. Answers

a. **True** – oedema also decreased.
b. **True**
c. **True**
d. **True** – also diabetes, steroids.
e. **False** – MRI is the most sensitive means of detection.

(Sutton pp1783–1784; Dähnert p257)

15. Answers

a. **True**
b. **True**
c. **True**
d. **True**
e. **True**

(Reeder p54)

16. Answers

- **a. False** – most are idiopathic.
- **b. False** – most common in the thoracolumbar spine.
- **c. False** – sagittal views are superior.
- **d. True**
- **e. False**

(Dähnert pp204–205)

17. Answers

- **a. True**
- **b. True**
- **c. True**
- **d. True**
- **e. True**

(Reeder p194)

18. Answers

- **a. True** – in 40% of degenerate discs.
- **b. False** – reduced.
- **c. False** – increases the thickness.
- **d. True**
- **e. True**

(Saifuddin A, Blease S, MacSweeney E. Axial loaded MRI of the lumbar spine. *Clin Radiol* 2003;58:661–671)

19. Answers

- **a. True**
- **b. True**
- **c. True**
- **d. False** – causes generalised sclerosis.
- **e. False** – focal sclerosis occurs.

(Reeder p212)

20. Answers

- **a. False** – a single level is involved in 75%.
- **b. True**
- **c. False** – disc space and vertebral enhancement occurs.
- **d. False** – MRI is more sensitive.
- **e. True**

(Dähnert p202; Haaga et al. pp806–808)

21. Answers

- **a. True**
- **b. False** – hyperparathyroidism.
- **c. False**
- **d. True**
- **e. True**

(Chapman & Nakielny 2003 p391)

22. Answers

- **a. True** – secondary to exophthalmos.
- **b. True** – can also cause a small orbit due to orbital dysplasia.
- **c. False** – the orbit and optic canal are small, due to bony encroachment.
- **d. False** – small orbit.
- **e. True**

(Reeder p103)

23. Answers

- **a. True** – the majority occur following penetrating trauma.
- **b. True** – palsies of all nerves passing through the cavernous sinus may be seen.
- **c. True**
- **d. False** – drainage via cortical veins is rare.
- **e. False** – treat by embolisation with detachable balloons, or coils.

(Haaga et al. p460; Dähnert p338)

24. Answers

- **a. True** – due to phleboliths.
- **b. True**
- **c. True**
- **d. True** – due to myositis ossificans and phthisis bulbis.
- **e. False**

(Reeder p114)

25. Answers

- **a. False** – trapped but not organified.
- **b. False** – no significant salivary excretion occurs, so saliva does not need to be cleared, unlike with pertechnetate.
- **c. True** – or high resolution, converging.
- **d. False** – 20 minutes.
- **e. True** – also IV.

(Chapman & Nakielny 2001 pp338–340)

26. Answers

- **a. False** – 98% are secondary.
- **b. True**
- **c. False** – no enhancement.
- **d. True**
- **e. False** – causes sigmoid sinus thrombosis.

(Dähnert pp375–376)

27. Answers

- **a. False** – frontal in 60%, ethmoids next commonest at 30%.
- **b. True** – this does not occur with sinusitis.
- **c. True**
- **d. False** – thin rim enhancement occurs.
- **e. True** – secondary to debris and fungal material.

(Dähnert pp385–386)

28. Answers

a. **True** – types IIA and IIB.
b. **False** – low reflectivity.
c. **True**
d. **False** – lateral aspects of the superior two-thirds, where the highest concentration of C-cells are.
e. **True**

(Ahuja & Evans pp48–49)

29. Answers

a. **True**
b. **False** – biopsy is contraindicated.
c. **True**
d. **False** – enhancement occurs early, immediately after injection.
e. **True**

(Sutton pp1492–1493; Dähnert p381)

30. Answers

a. **True**
b. **False** – rare.
c. **True** – 95% are found below the inferior border.
d. **False** – thin-walled.
e. **True** – 90% are hypervascular.

(Ahuja & Evans p59)

Module Six: Examination Three – Questions

1. **The following are true of the coils involved in MRI scanning:**

   a. shim coils are used to send RF pulses.
   b. gradient coils can be used for 'spoiling' in gradient echo.
   c. a head coil both transmits and receives RF signals.
   d. surface coils are cooled by liquid helium.
   e. quadrature coils increase SNR by a factor of four.

2. **Regarding the anatomy of the spine:**

   a. the intervertebral disc forms a secondary cartilaginous joint.
   b. the facet joints are synovial.
   c. the vertebral column ossifies in membrane.
   d. the posterior longitudinal ligament attaches to the vertebral bodies.
   e. the L5 nerve root exits beneath the L4 pedicle.

3. **Concerning the skull:**

   a. the diploic space contains marrow.
   b. diploic veins communicate with the dural venous sinuses.
   c. the anterior clinoid processes arise from the greater wing of sphenoid.
   d. the calvarium ossifies in cartilage.
   e. periosteum is only found on the outer surfaces.

4. **When imaging cerebral blood flow with SPECT:**

   a. 500 MBq of ^{99m}Tc-HMPAO is a suitable dose.
   b. ^{99m}Tc-HMPAO crosses the blood–brain barrier.
   c. ^{99m}Tc-HMPAO shows minimal redistribution following injection.
   d. imaging is performed with the patient supine.
   e. in patients with epilepsy, imaging should be delayed until the interictal period.

5. **Meningiomas:**

   a. are supratentorial in over 80%.
   b. cause hyperostosis of the adjacent skull.
   c. are frequently of increased attenuation at unenhanced CT.
   d. cause enlargement of vascular grooves in the skull vault.
   e. show an enhancing 'tail' of dura at MRI.

6. **Regarding pituitary adenomas:**

    a. most are microadenomas.
    b. macroadenomas often calcify.
    c. microadenomas enhance with gadolinium at MRI.
    d. pituitary apoplexy is a frequent complication of a macroadenoma.
    e. inferior petrosal sinus sampling has a diagnostic accuracy of 95% for corticotrophic adenomas.

7. **In HIV-positive patients, cerebral toxoplasmosis:**

    a. usually presents with headache.
    b. causes solitary lesions in the majority.
    c. results in a diffuse leptomeningitis.
    d. calcifies following treatment.
    e. rarely involves the basal ganglia.

8. **Osmotic myelinolysis:**

    a. is most common in chronic alcoholics.
    b. commonly affects only the pons.
    c. does not cause abnormalities at CT.
    d. results in high signal in the pons at T2-weighted MRI.
    e. causes cerebellar white matter lesions.

9. **Regarding the diagnosis of ischaemic stroke with MRI:**

    a. acutely ischaemic areas are bright on diffusion-weighted images.
    b. diffusion-weighted (DW) MRI is abnormal within 6 hours.
    c. after 2 weeks, DW MRI shows the infarct as a low signal area.
    d. gyral contrast enhancement can persist for up to 12 months.
    e. abnormalities are less extensive on perfusion-weighted than DW images.

10. **The following are features of cerebral cavernous angiomas:**

    a. intense enhancement following IV contrast in the majority.
    b. a low signal rim at T2-weighted MRI.
    c. large feeding vessels at MRI.
    d. a 'mulberry' appearance at MRI.
    e. focal neurological deficits as the commonest presentation.

11. **Bilateral signal abnormalities in the thalami occur in:**

    a. variant Creutzfeldt–Jakob disease.
    b. carbon monoxide poisoning.
    c. Leigh's disease.
    d. hypoxic brain injury.
    e. Japanese encephalitis.

12. Cerebral aneurysms:

a. occur in the anterior circulation in most cases.
b. are usually of increased density at unenhanced CT.
c. are commonly multiple.
d. of 2 mm are detected by MRA with a sensitivity of 90–95%.
e. treated with GDC coils are a contraindication to subsequent MRI.

13. Regarding malignant disease of the meninges:

a. serial lumbar punctures are more sensitive than contrast-enhanced MRI.
b. dural carcinomatosis is most often due to breast cancer.
c. leptomeningeal carcinomatosis does not follow the gyral contours.
d. leptomeningeal metastases usually present with headache.
e. calcification is a common finding.

14. Craniopharyngiomas:

a. originate from remnants of Rathke's cleft.
b. are often completely solid lesions.
c. demonstrate contrast enhancement at CT.
d. are typically hypervascular at angiography.
e. commonly contain calcification at CT.

15. The following are intracranial features of neurofibromatosis type 1:

a. meningiomas as the commonest finding.
b. hydrocephalus.
c. 'moyamoya' appearance at arteriography.
d. spontaneously regressing hamartomas.
e. foci of white matter high signal at T2-weighted MRI.

16. Regarding spinal dysraphisms:

a. spina bifida occulta is associated with lipomeningocoele.
b. most are of the spina bifida occulta subtype.
c. spina bifida aperta is associated with neurological deficits in over 90% of cases.
d. a butterfly vertebra is due to a failure of fusion of the lateral halves of the vertebral body.
e. coronal clefts usually occur in the lower cervical spine.

17. Following lumbar discectomy, scar tissue can be differentiated from residual or recurrent disc herniation by:

a. mass effect.
b. thecal retraction toward the soft tissue mass.
c. early homogeneous enhancement.
d. radicular pain.
e. a smooth margin.

18. Regarding endplate changes in degenerative disease:

a. type I change results in low signal at T1-weighted MRI.
b. type II change can be demonstrated at CT.
c. fatty change is the commonest form.
d. most patients with type II change eventually progress to type III.
e. type III change is of high signal at T2-weighted MRI.

19. A narrowed interpedicular distance may be due to:

a. Marfan's syndrome.
b. acromegaly.
c. myelomeningocoele.
d. Klippel–Feil syndrome.
e. diastematomyelia.

20. With respect to syringomyelia:

a. it is most common in the thoracic spinal cord.
b. the cord is frequently enlarged at the level of the syrinx.
c. it is associated with cerebellar ectopia in most cases.
d. flow void occurs at spin echo MRI.
e. the syrinx does not fill with contrast at CT myelography.

21. Regarding adamantinomas:

a. the majority arise from dentigerous cysts.
b. they are usually found in the maxilla.
c. there is an association with an impacted tooth.
d. they commonly occur around puberty.
e. scalloped margins and cortical expansion are typical.

22. At MRI, enlargement of the optic nerve may be due to:

a. multiple sclerosis.
b. sarcoid.
c. neurofibromatosis.
d. optic nerve glioma.
e. acromegaly.

23. **If, at CT, the lacrimal glands are enlarged, causes include:**

   a. Wegener's granulomatosis.
   b. syphilis.
   c. mumps.
   d. lymphoma.
   e. thyroid eye disease.

24. **Concerning thyroid eye disease:**

   a. unilateral proptosis occurs.
   b. lateral rectus is the most frequently involved muscle.
   c. swelling is confined to the belly of the extra-ocular muscles.
   d. muscles show increased signal at T1 weighted MRI.
   e. the extraconal fat undergoes atrophy.

25. **The following are true of magnetic resonance angiography (MRA):**

   a. time-of-flight (TOF) MRA is most sensitive to flow in the plane of the slice.
   b. 2-dimensional has superior resolution to 3-dimensional TOF-MRA.
   c. TOF-MRA is sensitive to slow flow.
   d. phase-contrast (PC) MRA can measure flow velocity.
   e. PC-MRA is sensitive to in-plane flow.

26. **The following are common CT signs of malignant otitis externa:**

   a. soft tissue density in external auditory canal.
   b. fluid-filled mastoid.
   c. obliteration of fat planes beneath the temporal bone.
   d. bone erosion of the clivus.
   e. intracranial extension of disease.

27. **Causes of maxillary sinus opacification with bone destruction include:**

   a. mucormycosis.
   b. Wegener's granulomatosis.
   c. acute sinusitis.
   d. maxillary dentigerous cyst.
   e. blow-out fracture of the orbit.

28. **Regarding US of the multinodular thyroid:**

   a. it is the commonest pathological condition of the thyroid.
   b. calcification is seen in 40–60%.
   c. solid nodules are predominantly of low reflectivity.
   d. a 'comet tail' sign is seen.
   e. a cystic component is present in 10–30%.

29. **Concerning malignant tumours of the larynx:**

a. carcinoma of the true cords is the commonest type.
b. supraglottic tumours are best assessed with CT.
c. invasion of the laryngeal cartilage is best seen at CT.
d. soft tissue involvement is best seen at MRI.
e. lymphomas are best seen at fat-suppressed MRI.

30. **Glomus jugulare tumours:**

a. extend intracranially.
b. present with tinnitus.
c. enhance intensely.
d. cause destruction of the auditory ossicles.
e. splay the internal and external carotid arteries.

Module Six: Examination Three – Answers

1. Answers

a. **False** – used to improve homogeneity of the main field, B_0.
b. **True**
c. **True**
d. **False**
e. **False** – by a factor of $\sqrt{2}$.

(Westbrook & Kaut pp224–229; Hashemi & Bradley p28)

2. Answers

a. **True**
b. **True**
c. **False** – ossifies in cartilage.
d. **False** – PLL attaches to the discs, but is separated from the vertebra by the basivertebral veins.
e. **False** – beneath the L5 pedicle.

(Butler et al. pp304–326)

3. Answers

a. **True**
b. **True**
c. **False** – lesser wing of sphenoid.
d. **False** – ossifies in membrane.
e. **False**

(Butler et al. pp19–25)

4. Answers

a. **True**
b. **True**
c. **True**
d. **True**
e. **False** – ictal imaging is more sensitive than interictal.

(Chapman & Nakielny 2001 pp297–300)

5. Answers

a. **True**
b. **True** – this is not related to tumour size.
c. **True** – 60–75% are of increased attenuation (40–50 HU).
d. **True**
e. **True** – this is not pathognomonic, it also occurs with metastases and schwannomas.

(Grainger & Allison pp2336–2337; Haaga et al. pp166–168)

6. Answers

a. **False** – 70–80% are macroadenomas.
b. **False** – rare.
c. **False** – no enhancement with gadolinium.
d. **False** – rarely occurs.
e. **True**

(Dähnert pp264–266)

7. Answers

a. **True** – also with confusion and personality change.
b. **False** – multiple lesions are typical.
c. **False** – focal leptomeningitis occurs adjacent to cerebral lesions.
d. **True** – rarely.
e. **False** – the basal ganglia are frequently affected.

(Grainger & Allison pp2383–2384)

8. Answers

a. **True**
b. **True**
c. **False** – low attenuation in the pons may be seen.
d. **True**
e. **True**

(Dähnert p265)

9. Answers

a. **True** – but dark on maps of apparent diffusion coefficient (ADC).
b. **True**
c. **True** – due to increased mobility of water protons in areas of gliosis.
d. **True**
e. **False** – more extensive, showing both infarct and ischaemic penumbra.

(Grainger & Allison pp2353–2356)

10. Answers

a. **False** – enhancement is often absent or minimal.
b. **True** – due to haemosiderin and ferritin from previous haemorrhage.
c. **False** – this is a feature of arteriovenous malformation.
d. **True**
e. **False** – seizures are the commonest presentation.

(Grainger & Allison p2371; Haaga et al. pp297–298; Dähnert p266)

11. Answers

a. **True** – high signal in the pulvinar at T2-weighting.
b. **True**
c. **True**
d. **True**
e. **True**

(Chapman & Nakielny 2003 p438)

12. Answers

a. **True** – 80–90% are located in the anterior circulation.
b. **True**
c. **False** – only 20% are multiple.
d. **False** – the sensitivity is 77–94% for aneurysms > 5 mm, and worse for smaller aneurysms.
e. **False** – not a contraindication, although image quality is degraded in the area of the coils.

(Grainger & Allison pp2366–2369; Haaga et al. pp289–291)

13. Answers

a. **True** – and in turn, MRI is more sensitive than CT.
b. **True** – also lymphoma, prostate and neuroblastoma.
c. **False** – enhancement follows the brain surface.
d. **True**
e. **False**

(Grainger & Allison p234; Haaga et al. pp198–199)

14. Answers

a. **True**
b. **False** – most are partially cystic.
c. **True**
d. **False** – avascular.
e. **True**

(Dähnert p272)

15. Answers

a. **False** – optic gliomas are the commonest feature, seen in 30% of cases.
b. **True** – due to aqueductal stenosis or tectal/tegmental tumours.
c. **True**
d. **True** – hamartomas appear from 3 years of age and regress in adolescence.
e. **True** – most common in pons, cerebellum and splenium of corpus callosum.

(Dähnert p310; Herron J, Darrah R, Quaghebeur G. Intracranial manifestations of the neurocutaneous syndromes. *Clin Radiol* 2000;55:82–98)

16. Answers

a. **True**
b. **False** – spina bifida aperta comprises 85% of all cases.
c. **True**
d. **True**
e. **False** – lower thoracic and lumbar spine.

(Dähnert pp180–181)

17. Answers

a. **False** – scar and disc may show mass effect.
b. **True** – more common with scar.
c. **True** – a feature of scar.
d. **False** – disc and scar both cause radicular pain.
e. **True** – disc shows a smooth margin, scar tends to be more irregular.

(Babar S, Saifuddin A. MRI of the post-discectomy lumbar spine. *Clin Radiol* 2002;57:969–981)

18. Answers

a. **True** – due to marrow oedema.
b. **False** – only type III (sclerotic) changes are visible at CT.
c. **True**
d. **False** – type II change is usually stable.
e. **False** – low signal at T1 and T2 weighting.

(Dähnert p200; Haaga et al. p737)

19. Answers

a. **False** – widened.
b. **True**
c. **False** – widened.
d. **True**
e. **False** – increased interpedicular distance.

(Reeder pp220–221)

20. Answers

a. **False** – most common in the cervical cord.
b. **True** – enlarged in 80%, atrophic in 10% and normal in 10%.
c. **True**
d. **True** – due to CSF pulsation.
e. **False** – delayed filling at 4–8 hours occurs.

(Dähnert pp220–221; Grainger & Allison p2345)

21. Answers

a. **False** – most arise from enamel type epithelial tissue around the tooth; one third arise from dentigerous cysts.
b. **False** – 75% found on the mandible.
c. **True**
d. **False** – 4th to 5th decade.
e. **True**

(Dähnert p177)

22. Answers

a. **True** – due to optic neuritis.
b. **True**
c. **True**
d. **True**
e. **False** – extra-ocular muscles are enlarged, however.

(Reeder pp110–111)

23. Answers

a. **True**
b. **True**
c. **True**
d. **True**
e. **True**

(Reeder p116)

24. Answers

a. **True** – in 30%, but it is usually bilateral.
b. **False** – inferior rectus and medial rectus are most often affected.
c. **True** – the anterior tendon is not involved.
d. **True** – due to fatty infiltration.
e. **False** – both the intra- and extra-conal fat hypertrophies.

(Grainger & Allison pp2529–2530)

25. Answers

a. **False** – in-plane saturation occurs, it is most sensitive to flow perpendicular to the slice.
b. **False** – resolution is superior with 3D TOF-MRA.
c. **True**
d. **True**
e. **True**

(Westbrook & Kaut pp186–199)

26. Answers

a. **True** – seen in 100%.
b. **True**
c. **True**
d. **False** – seen in 9%.
e. **False** – present in only 9%.

(Dähnert p385)

27. Answers

a. **True** – also aspergillosis, TB and syphilis.
b. **True**
c. **False** – no bone destruction.
d. **False** – no bone destruction.
e. **True**

(Dähnert p351)

28. Answers

a. **True**
b. **False** – 25%.
c. **False** – mainly isoreflective to normal gland.
d. **True**
e. **False** – 60%.

(Ahuja & Evans p53)

29. Answers

- a. **True**
- b. **False** – endoscopy is the best means of assessment.
- c. **True**
- d. **True**
- e. **True**

(Sutton pp1498–1499)

30. Answers

- a. **True**
- b. **True**
- c. **True**
- d. **True**
- e. **False** – this is a feature of carotid body tumours.

(Dähnert pp387–389)

References

Ahuja A, Evans R, eds. (2000). *Practical Head and Neck Ultrasound.* Greenwich Medical Media, London.

Allan PL, Dubbins PA, Pozniak MA, McDicken WN. (2000). *Clinical Doppler Ultrasound.* Churchill Livingstone, London.

Bates J, ed. (1997). *Practical Gynaecological Ultrasound.* Greenwich Medical Media, London.

Baxter GM, Allan PLP, Morley P, eds. (1999). *Clinical Diagnostic Ultrasound.* 2nd edn. Blackwell Science, Oxford.

Bell G, Findlay D. (1986). *Basic Radiographic Positioning and Anatomy.* Baillière Tindall, London.

Brant W, Helms CA, eds. (1999). *Fundamentals of Diagnostic Radiology*, 2nd edn. Saunders, Philadelphia.

Butler P, Mitchell AWM, Ellis H, eds. (1999). *Applied Radiological Anatomy.* Cambridge University Press, Cambridge.

Chapman S, Nakielny R. (2001). *A Guide to Radiological Procedures.* 4th edn. WB Saunders, London.

Chapman S, Nakielny R. (2003). *Aids to Radiological Differential Diagnosis.* 4th edn. WB Saunders, London.

Dähnert W. (2002). *Radiology Review Manual.* 5th edn. Lippincott Williams & Wilkins, Baltimore.

Dendy PP, Heaton B. (1999). *Physics for Diagnostic Radiology.* 2nd edn. Institute of Physics Publishing, Bristol.

Dewbury K, Meire H, Cosgrove D, Farrant P, eds. (2000). *Clinical Ultrasound: A Comprehensive Text.* 2nd edn. Churchill Livingstone, London.

Farr RF, Allisy-Roberts PJ. (1998). *Physics for Medical Imaging.* WB Saunders, London.

Francis IS, Aviv RI, Dick EA. (1999). *Fundamental Aspects of Radiology.* Remedica, London.

Grainger RG, Allison DJ, Adam A, Dixon AK, eds. (2001). *Grainger & Allison's Diagnostic Radiology: A Textbook of Medical Imaging.* 4th edn. Churchill Livingstone, London.

Haaga JR, Lanzieri CF, Gilkeson RC, eds. (2002). *CT and MR Imaging of the Whole Body.* 4th edn. Mosby, St. Louis.

Harris JH, Harris W, eds. (2000). *The Radiology of Emergency Medicine.* 4th edn. Lippincott Williams & Wilkins, Baltimore.

Hashemi RH, Bradley WG. (1997). *MRI: The Basics.* Lippincott Williams & Wilkins, Baltimore.

Husband JE, Reznek RH, eds. (1998). *Imaging in Oncology.* Martin Dunitz, London.

Reeder MM. (2003). *Reeder & Felson's Gamuts in Radiology: Comprehensive Lists of Roentgen Differential Diagnosis.* 4th edn. Springer, New York.

Rogers LF. (2002). *The Radiology of Skeletal Trauma.* 3rd edn. Churchill Livingstone, Philadelphia.

Ryan S, McNicholas M. (1994). *Anatomy for Diagnostic Imaging.* Saunders, London.

Sutton D, ed. (2002). *Textbook of Radiology and Imaging.* 7th edn. Churchill Livingstone, London.
Westbrook C, Kaut C. (1998). *MRI in Practice.* 2nd edn. Blackwell Science, London.